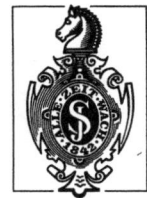

Rainer Ch. Otto   Josef Wellauer

Ultrasound-Guided Biopsy and Drainage

With Contributions by
G. Pedio, H. R. Burger, H. J. Einighammer,
and R. Hauke

Translated by Terry C. Telger

With 91 Illustrations

Springer-Verlag
Berlin Heidelberg New York Tokyo

Professor Dr. med. RAINER CH. OTTO (Leitender Arzt)
Professor Dr. med. JOSEF WELLAUER (Direktor)
Röntgendiagnostisches Zentralinstitut
Universitätsspital Zürich
Rämistraße 100
CH-8091 Zürich

Translator:

TERRY C. TELGER
6112 Waco Way
Ft. Worth, TX 76133
USA

Title of the original German edition:
Ultraschallgeführte Biopsie (Series: *Die Radiologische Klinik*) by R. Ch. Otto,
J. Wellauer
© Springer-Verlag Berlin Heidelberg 1985

ISBN-13:978-3-642-70991-3   e-ISBN-13:978-3-642-70989-0
DOI: 10.1007/978-3-642-70989-0

2121/3130-543210

Table of Contents

List of Contributors

BURGER, H. R., Dr. med., Oberarzt, Institut für Pathologie, Universität Zürich, Schmelzbergstraße 12, CH-8091 Zürich

EINIGHAMMER, H. J., Dipl. Phys., Dr. rer. nat., Neurologische Universitätsklinik, Moorenstraße 5, D-4000 Düsseldorf

HAUKE, R., Dipl., Phys., Dr. rer. nat., Gesellschaft für Medizin. Techn. Informationssysteme, Marienstraße 2, D-7910 Neu-Ulm

PEDIO, G., Professor Dr. med., Leitender Arzt, Abteilung für Zytologie, Institut für Pathologie, Universitätsspital, CH-8091 Zürich

"... so it is not good for men to fear all that is not already known and settled, and thus feel that it is bad and harmful to strive for a greater perfection than already exists."

Hölderlin to his mother, 16. November 1799

A. Introduction

1 General

The modern cross-sectional imaging methods of sonography and computed tomography, developed in the early 1970s, have contributed greatly to noninvasive studies of the parenchymatous organs and permit the evaluation of pathologic changes in areas that were previously accessible only to invasive, indirect, or inadequate examination.

Today these imaging methods have reached a very high level of refinement and are available not only in large centers but also in many smaller clinics and consulting rooms, enabling patients to derive maximum benefit from them. Recently, sonography and computed tomography have been joined by yet another cross-sectional imaging modality known as nuclear magnetic resonance, which operates without X-rays and can generate high-resolution tomograms in various planes.

Physicians can now rapidly establish a diagnosis in many patients with the aid of these modern imaging techniques. If the images are not immediately diagnostic, they can still guide the physician in selecting further investigations that are likely to be of very great benefit in identifying the underlying disease process.

As in conventional radiography, many lesions that are detected with the newer imaging methods will require microscopic tissue analysis before a definitive treatment can be chosen. This particularly applies to neoplastic diseases, in which it is important not only to localize the lesion but also to establish its nature, since accurate staging and grading of the tumor are prerequisite to formulating an appropriate plan of treatment and making an accurate prognosis.

Everyday experience confirms the difficulty of identifying a focal lesion in an organ as being malignant or benign. After the introduction of sonography and computed tomography, it soon became apparent that these studies would have to be supplemented by percutaneous biopsy and specimen collection so that the previously detected mass or area of abnormality could be subjected to microscopic or bacteriologic study prior to institution of treatment.

The routine use of operative exposure should be rejected as too invasive in view of the prevalence of benign or possibly congenital structural anomalies and simple anatomic variants.

Biopsy methods suitable for routine diagnostic use must satisfy several criteria:

1. They must not expose the patient to excessive risk.
2. They must be highly accurate and reproducible.
3. They must yield material that is useful for cytologic, histologic, and bacteriologic evaluation and will enable the specialist to make an accurate diagnosis.

"Blind" biopsy without benefit of continuous visual control has an unacceptably high failure rate and can be hazardous depending on the type of needle used and the area biopsied. It may be appropriate in larger organs when there is suspicion of diffuse parenchymatous disease, but it has no place in the evaluation of deeply situated focal lesions.

Intraoperative biopsy, as practiced in the pancreas, for example, can be useful in the evaluation of inflammatory or malignant masses whose exact nature is not grossly apparent. False-negative findings are not uncommon with pancreatic tumors, for the needle may miss the tumor focus under palpation alone and enter a surrounding area of pancreatitis. If surgery is undertaken, a wedge excision will usually provide sufficient material for histologic examination, and needle biopsy will not be required.

Needle biopsy of the lung under fluoroscopic control in one or two planes has become a standard procedure that is practiced at many centers. Its risks are negligible when the proper technique is observed [117, 156, 157].

Needle biopsy of the retroperitoneal lymph nodes *after lymphography* has not become widely accepted.

Since 1977/1978, we have been able to perform *ultrasound-guided fine-needle aspirations* under continuous visual control using a linear-array transducer with a central aperture that was developed at our institute in cooperation with Japanese engineers (Toshiba). This technique provides a very good diagnostic yield at low risk and is routinely practiced at our clinic and at many other centers [126, 127].

We also perform biopsies under *computed tomographic guidance*, which, despite the greater effort and cost involved, is extremely useful in biopsies of very small lesions that are not easily delineated by ultrasound.

Even in biopsies of diffuse parenchymatous diseases such as glomerulonephritis and hepatic cirrhosis, cross-sectional imaging is still recommended for guiding the procedure. Tissue retrieval is more certain, the biopsy site can be precisely monitored, and the inadvertent puncture of blood vessels can be avoided.

Recently, increasing attention has been given to certain percutaneous *therapeutic procedures* that require visual control. The introduction of drainage tubes into hollow organs (nephrostomy) or abscesses with palliative or curative intent is now possible with a high degree of accuracy and can sometimes obviate the need for operative intervention under general anesthesia. If the puncture is unsuccessful, the surgeon can still operate and help the patient by "conventional" means. It must be remembered, of course, that even the insertion of a small-caliber needle is an invasive procedure, and complications cannot be ruled out with certainty. Hence the selection of patients for diagnostic or therapeutic puncture should be based on far stricter criteria than are applied to macromorphological examinations.

2 Historical Development of Aspiration Biopsy Under Ultrasound and Computed Tomographic Guidance

2.1 Cross-Sectional Imaging Methods

Sonography

Fluoroscopic methods were first used in the 1930s for the localization and aspiration of deep-seated lesions [11]. Owing in part to this technical advance, diagnostic cytology assumed an ever-increasing importance, becoming a major tool at large oncologic centers [180].

Ultrasonography was first introduced in to medicine by Dussik, who in 1937 used ultrasound waves to demonstrate the intracranial extent of cerebral tumors [28]. He called his method "hyperphonography of the brain" and claimed that it had both diagnostic and therapeutic value [29].

After World War II, initial experiments were done on the use of ultrasound for examinations of intraabdominal organs [100, 175], building on theoretical groundwork laid down earlier [135]. It was not until the 1970s that ultrasound came to be used widely and routinely for imaging of the abdomen, extraabdominal soft structures, and heart [31, 37, 89, 137]. Reports on the first ultrasound-guided fine-needle aspirations were also published in the early 1970s [52, 73].

Soon, fine-gauge needles like the Chiba needle were being used in the United States and Scandinavia in conjunction with static scanners for ultrasound-guided aspiration biopsies of space-occupying lesions [18, 52, 91]. From there it was a short step to the performance of biopsies under real-time conditions, though initially this method posed serious technical difficulties that limited its general acceptance [73, 101].

During the period from 1976 to 1977, a procedure was developed at the Department of Diagnostic Radiology of Zurich University Clinic in collaboration with Japanese engineers that enabled tissue specimens to be collected from deep within the body under real-time sonographic control. This technique was decidedly superior to methods previously available, including biopsy under computed tomographic guidance [122, 123, 126].

Continuous visual monitoring of the needle tip throughout the biopsy procedure offers three important advantages:

1. All structures that lie in the path of the biopsy needle can be identifed as the needle is advanced and can continue to be monitored after the needle is withdrawn.

2. Complications, especially significant hemorrhage, can be recognized as they arise.
3. The needle can be guided safely and accurately to the area of diagnostic interest. Fine-needle aspiration biopsy under continuous ultrasound guidance is the only technique that provides a high yield of diagnostically useful material from sites deep within the body.

Since its introduction, various authors have adopted and in some cases modified the technique of aspiration biopsy under real-time ultrasound guidance [23, 42, 66, 71, 87, 114], and application of the technique is expanding.

Computed Tomography

The principle of computed tomography was described in the early 1970s by Hounsfield [74], who also designed the first diagnostic instrument. A short time later percutaneous biopsies were being performed under computed tomographic guidance, but it was learned that, even with large focal masses, macromorphological findings were generally insufficient for an accurate interpretation [3, 64].

2.2 Cytology

The idea of using a thin needle to aspirate representative cells that would allow tumors to be diagnosed by histologic analysis without surgical intervention is not new. The concept was suggested as early as 1912 by Hirschfeld [68] and in 1913 by Ward [168], and the subject was readdressed by various authors after 1920 [19, 38, 63, 103].

The true founder of clinical cytology, however, was the Berlin physiologist Johannes Muller. In his monograph *Über den feineren Bau und die Formen der krankhaften Geschwülste* (On the Fine Structure and Forms of Pathologic Tumors 1838), Müller presents the basic microscopic criteria that distinguish the cells of benign and malignant tumors and compares the features of sarcomas and carcinomas [115].

The Swiss pathologist Lebert was the first, in 1845, to describe the diagnostic aspiration of tumors [93], a procedure which he performed in Zurich and other cities. But it was not until the 1920s that this method was seriously tested, and in subsequent decades it gained a growing number of advocates. Fine-needle aspiration biopsy experienced its greatest upswing in the 1960s [45]. Aspiration biopsy was slow to develop initially, largely because histopathology had long been a successful and established science and usually provided more accurate results.

Hematologists were instrumental in advancing and popularizing diagnostic cytology, for they were already familiar with the aspiration biopsy of bone marrow. From Hirschfeld [68], Ward [168], and Guthrie [63], this line of development can be traced through Swiss scientists such as Stahel [163] and Moeschlin [113] to the contemporary cytologists Lopes-Cardozo [98] and Zajicek [181]. English-speaking pathologists and clinicians such as Martin [103], Stewart [104], and Coley [19] helped to broaden the indications for fine-needle aspiration early in its development.

2.3 Fine Needles for the Collection of Cytologic Specimens

Fine-needle aspiration biopsy did not gain general acceptance until a suitable and sufficiently "atraumatic" needle had been developed [34, 46, 116], and until modern, high-resolution imaging modalities made it rational to supplement macromorphological examinations by fine-needle biopsy. The success of this procedure, with its low risk and high diagnostic yield, was closely bound up with continual improvements in fine-tissue analysis, including electron microscopy, and it was natural that the demand for fine-needle aspiration biopsies should parallel these improvements.

The fine, highly elastic, stylet-armed needle of Franzen, which was later copied in Japan as the "Chiba needle" with an outer diameter of approximately 0.7 mm, was first developed in 1960 exclusively for the aspiration of cellular material from the prostate [46], and was modified by Otho et al. to provide a safer technique of percutaneous transhepatic cholangiography [121]. In Japan the needle was also used for the intraoperative cytologic evaluation of pancreatic tumors, as it carried a far smaller risk of pancreatitis and hemorrhage than the large needles previously used. Also, it was difficult to place the larger needles accurately within the tumor if palpatory findings were uncertain, which resulted in a higher rate of false-negative results.

Since the popularization of cytology, which has contributed much to the development of ultrasound- and computed-tomographic-guided biopsy techniques, various methods of obtaining the desired cellular material have been devised. Each has its advantages and disadvantages. In the present book we describe an ultrasound-guided method of percutaneous needle biopsy that has been successfully used in more than 3000 patients at our institute, provides a high diagnostic yield, and is relatively easy to learn.

B. Principles and Technique

1 Principles of Ultrasound-Guided Biopsy Under Continuous Vision

For biopsies under continuous sonographic and visual control, there are three different ways in which real-time monitoring can be accomplished, depending on how the needle is oriented with respect to the ultrasound beam or the imag-

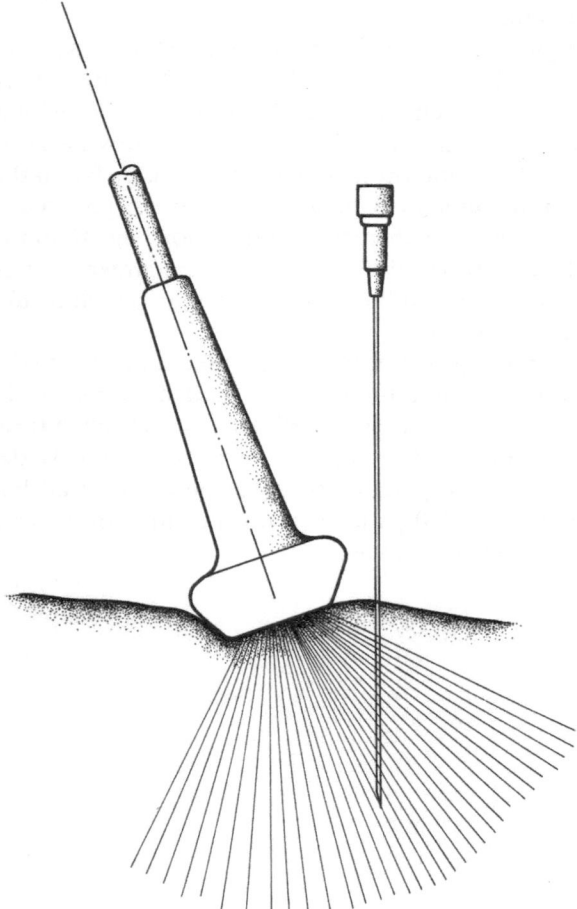

Fig. 1. "Freehand" biopsy under ultrasound control. The needle and transducer (here, a sector scanner) are not connected

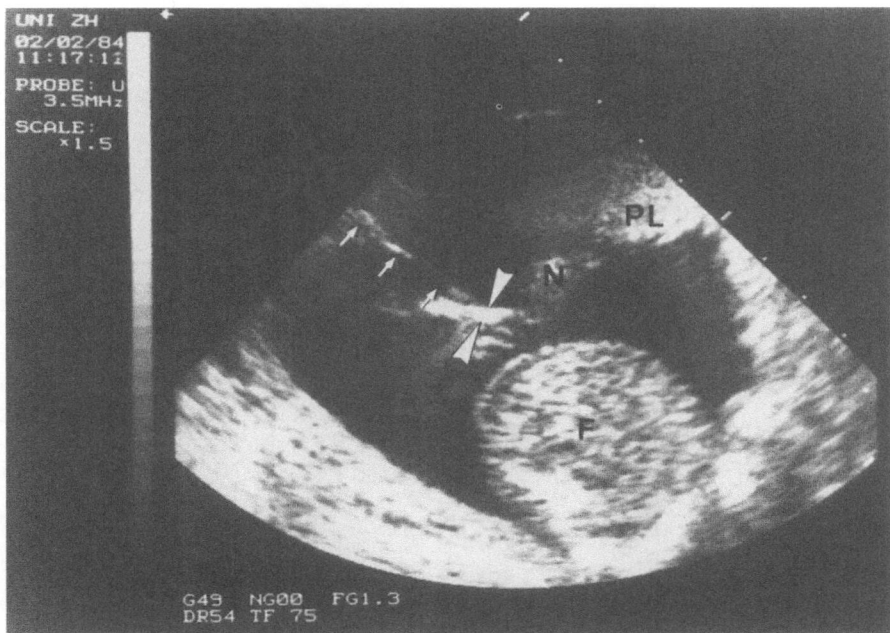

Fig. 2. Amniocentesis. A broad echo is seen at the tip of the amniocentesis needle *(large arrowheads)*. The needle is introduced into the amniotic cavity from the left *(small white arrows;* needle shaft; *F*, body of fetus; *PL*, placenta; *N*, umbilical cord)

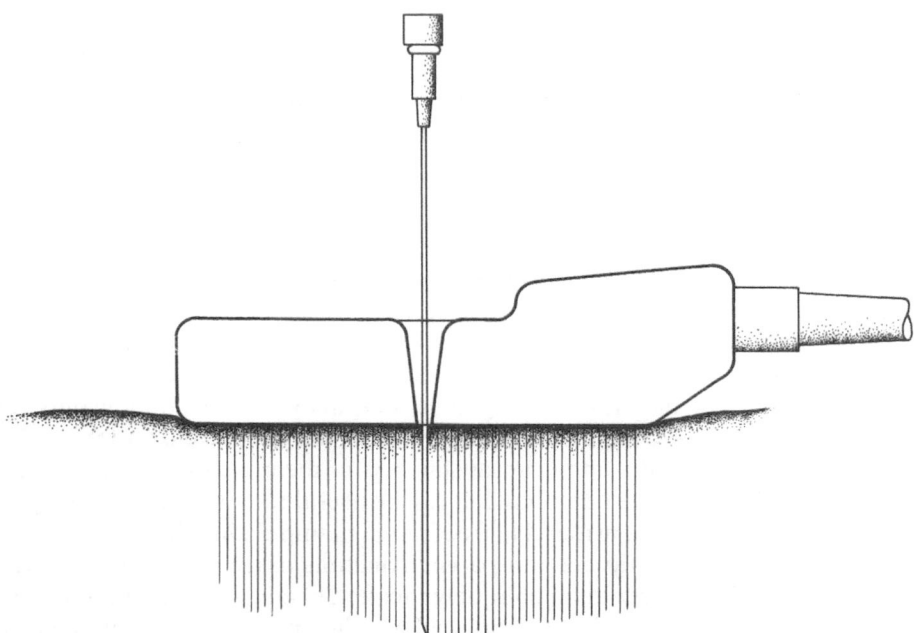

Fig. 3. Biopsy using a linear-array transducer with central aperture of the type developed in Zurich. The biopsy needle is advanced along the center of the sound field. The absence of crystal at the center creates a dark "sight line" on the monitor that designates the intended needle path

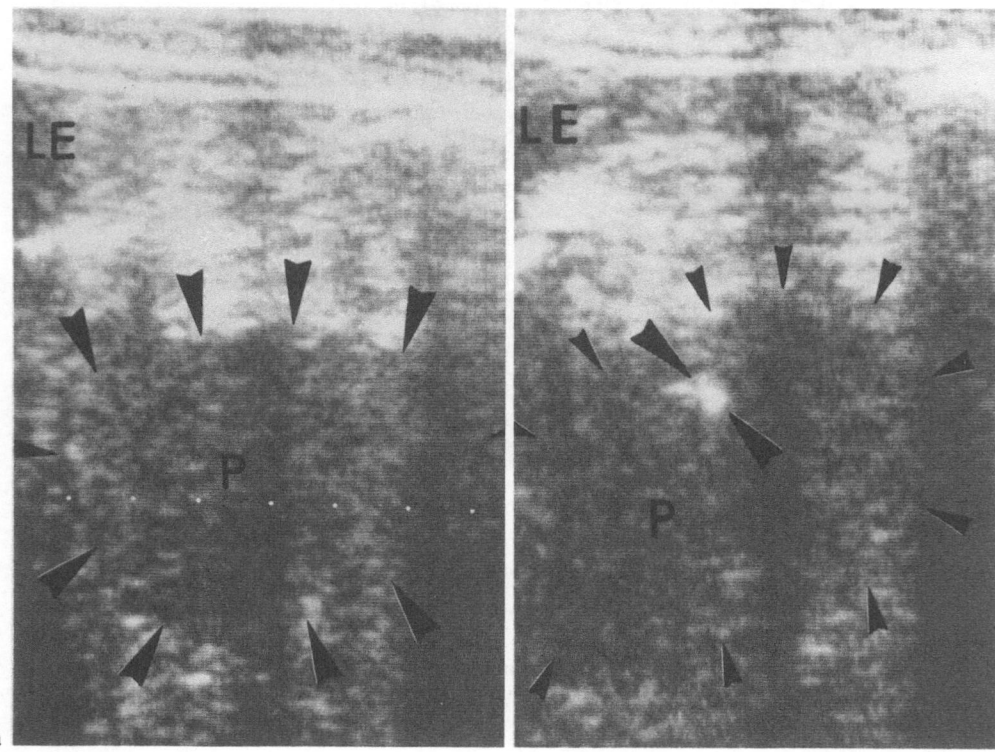

a

Fig. 4 a,b. Large pancreatic carcinoma *(P arrows). LE,* inferior margin of liver. **a** The sight line *(dark vertical line at center of image)* is faintly visible. The *white reference marks* are spaced approximately 1 cm apart. This image is typical of that seen on the monitor when the linear-array biopsy transducer is used. **b** Moment of tissue aspiration. The needle tip appears as a bright echo in the still-viable upper periphery of the tumor *(large arrows)*

ing plane of the transducer. The old practice of using a static scanner with a perforated biopsy transducer is too imprecise and is now considered obsolete.

The simplest monitoring method is to place the transducer onto the skin next to the puncture site and angle it as needed to localize the needle after insertion (Fig. 1). This method is appealing for its simplicity, but it is suitable only for selected applications. On the one hand, it requires the use of rigid and thus relatively large-gauge needles and is unsatisfactory for the puncture of solid space-occupying lesions. On the other hand, it can be useful for amniocentesis (Fig. 2) as it gives the operator considerable freedom in manipulating the needle.

Because the needle tip echo in parenchymatous tissue is usually reflected away from the transducer in an obliquely incident beam, localization of the biopsy needle can be very difficult. The weak needle tip echo in the oblique projection contrasts poorly with normal echoes returned from surrounding tissues.

8

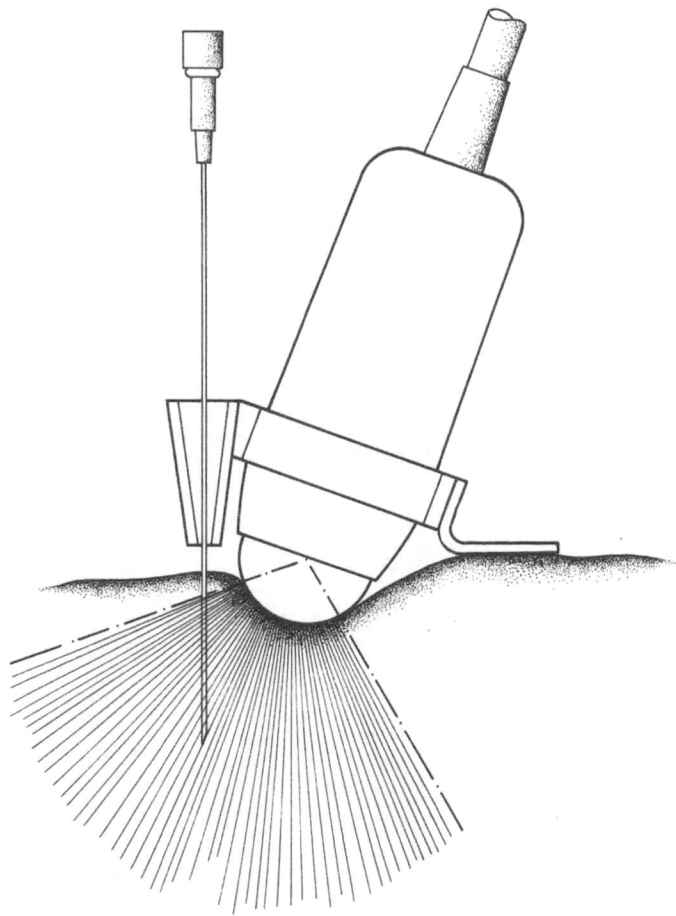

Fig. 5. Ultrasound-guided biopsy with a sector scanner. The needle and transducer are interconnected via a special needle guide. An electronic sight line on the monitor indicates the desired needle path

In the procedure developed in Zurich, which now exists in various modifications, the biopsy needle is inserted through an aperture in the center of the transducer (Fig. 3). It may be advanced into the body vertically or at a slightly oblique angle and remains visible throughout the procedure. Owing to the principle used, the tip of even a very thin needle produces a conspicuous echo, provided the axis of the needle coincides with the imaging plane of the transducer.

This guidance method also allows the use of fine, flexible needles, as represented by the Chiba needle. Such an instrument can easily be introduced vertically into the tissue without significant deviation from the desired path. If a flexible needle is advanced through tissue layers obliquely with respect to the transducer, deviation from a straight path is almost inevitable. On the other

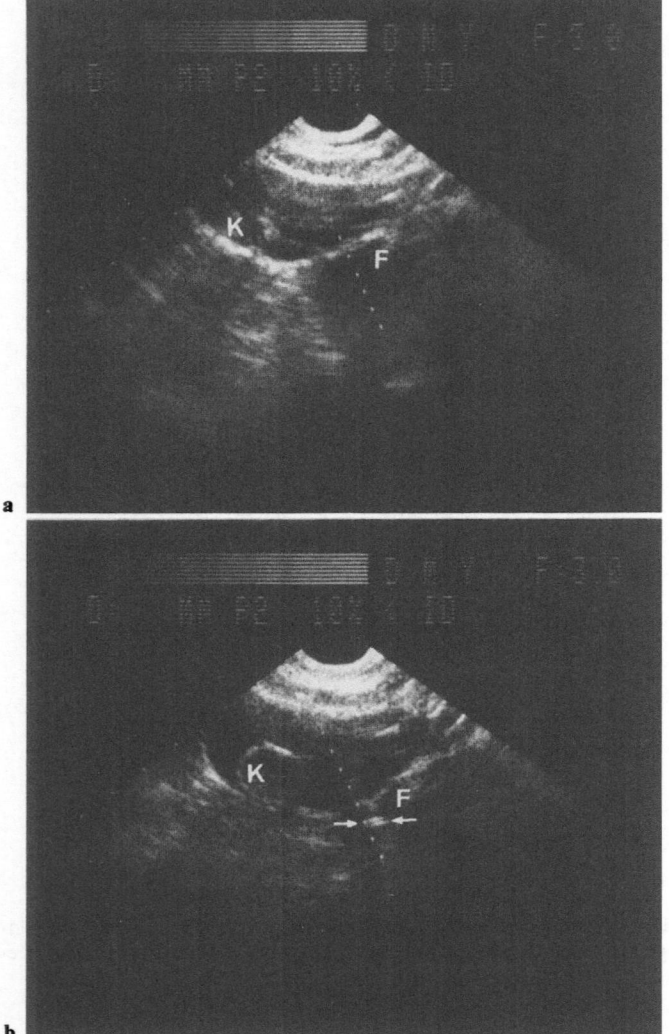

Fig. 6a,b. Transvesical follicular aspiration for collection of oocytes using the sector technique. *F*, follicle; *dotted line*, sight line for aspiration needle; *K*, bladder catheter cut obliquely by the beam. **a** Needle tip is not yet visible. **b** Needle tip at the center of the follicle (double echo marked with *two arrows*). The faintly visible needle shaft follows the dotted sight line from upper left to lower right

hand, a slight deviation of the needle tip from the tomographic plane can be adequately compensated by slight angular adjustment of the transducer.

Figure 4a,b illustrates the puncture of a large pancreatic carcinoma. The needle tip is visible as a bright echo at the upper (anterior), outer border of the tumor. Through visual control, the operator is able to insert the needle tip into the peripheral part of the tumor, which still contains viable tissue.

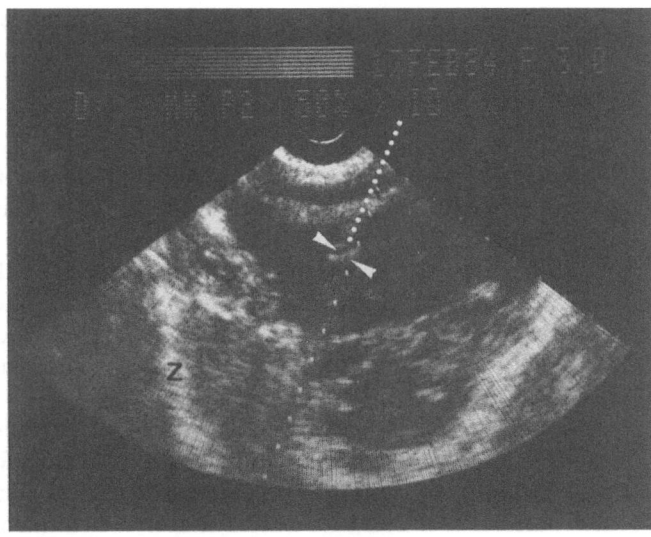

Fig. 7. Large hepatic abscess, seen as a hypoechoic mass extending far posteriorly. Fine-needle aspiration with a sector scanner *Arrows,* needle tip; shaft is marked by *closely spaced dots*; *Z,* diaphragm

Real-time sector scanners can also be used for biopsy guidance (Fig. 5). In this method the needle enters the image field obliquely and from the side, similary to the case in a free-hand biopsy. An electronic „sight line" on the sonographic image marks the intended path of needle insertion. This line must intersect the target to ensure that the needle tip will enter it when advanced.

We mainly use this procedure in follicular aspirations to collect oocytes for in vitro fertilization, especially since the sector scan technique is well suited for delineating the ovaries and other organs of the lesser pelvis. Figure 6 shows an example of this. The same procedure can be applied to aspirations of other hollow structures, such as dilated bile ducts, and of space-occupying lesions in the parenchymatous organs (Fig. 7).

Through experience, we have learned that a central needle insertion with a linear scanner is the most advantageous technique. Orientation is more easily accomplished than with an eccentric insertion, because the image field is only 8–10 cm wide. The path to the lesion is shorter and more direct than in the sector technique, and there is better resolution of deep echo structures.

2 Localizing the Biopsy Needle in the Sonographic Image

2.1 Preliminary Remarks

The earlier practice of localizing a suspicious focus with ultrasound, determining its depth, marking the entry site on the skin, and then advancing the needle blindly to the target has met with disfavor on account of its unacceptably high failure rate, even in biopsies of large masses. The simultaneous recording of an A-mode sonogram was helpful only in biopsies of cystic masses monitored with a static scanner. It soon became apparent that only continuous monitoring of the entire biopsy in real time would be able to lower the high failure rate and lessen the risk of the procedure.

When fine, highly elastic needles were used, monitoring with a transducer held next to the needle proved to be of little value except in aspirating of large fluid collections (e.g., amniocentesis). A fine needle can indeed reach a deep-seated soft-tissue lesion with little difficulty when introduced vertically, but the needle is then very difficult to localize with an obliquely incident beam. It was clear that the tomographic plane of the transducer and the axis of fine-needle insertion had to coincide exactly, both to minimize the length of the needle tract and to allow continuous monitoring of the needle during its insertion.

It had been determined empirically that when a needle was introduced vertically the tip was the part most likely to remain visible, and that this visibility varied with the shape and bevel of the tip and with certain tissue parameters (sound transmission through the skin, subcutaneous tissues, internal organs, etc.).

The phenomenon of needle tip echogenicity — one easily reproduced in water bath experiments — required further investigations of a physical nature both to elucidate the phenomenon and to identify the technically variable characteristics of the biopsy needle that related most closely to its brightness in sonograms. To date, very little research has been conducted in this area [69].

2.2 Physical Experiments and Considerations

H. J. EINIGHAMMER, R. HAUKE (pp.12-25)

Methods of Ultrasound-Guided Biopsy

Before discussing the direct localization of biopsy needles in the ultrasound image, we shall first mention „indirect" methods of biopsy guidance.

To illustrate the indirect method, let us assume that the operator is using a biopsy transducer of the formerly used type with a central needle guide and is unable to see the needle clearly on the screen of the A-scan device. First he must make a measurement to determine the distance of the target from the skin surface. Then he introduces the needle blindly to a preriously adjusted stop on the needle shaft, using the mechanical guide to ensure that the needle does not stray from the path of the beam. From the position of the end of the needle relative to the transducer, it is also possible to determine the presumptive location of the needle tip and mark it in the A-mode image. The procedure is similar for twodimensional B-scanners. In this case the presumptive needle tract is known because there is a rigid connection between the needle guide and transducer, and the position of the needle tip in the tract is easily determined when the needle length is known. If greater mobility of the biopsy needle is desired, the tip position can be measured in two coordinates by means of an articulated mechanism attached to the needle holder.

But even when such an arrangement is properly adjusted, there still exist two potential sources of error: first, the needle may bend as it is advanced; and second, local deviations of the sound velocity from the assumed mean value caused by local accumulations of fat can give a false distance measurement and also distort the B-mode image as a result of refraction, so that a discrepancy arises between mechanical and acoustic data [69, 81].

In the *direct* method of ultrasound guidance, the needle and tissue are imaged jointly as a common object. Thus, the position of the needle in the tissue is always accurately displayed, even if there is bowing of the needle or if there are variations of sound propagation velocity. Of course, the latter will still produce image distortions, but these will affect the tissue and needle equally. A disadvantage of the direct method is that the visibility of the needle tip deteriorates under unfavorable conditions (highly echogenic tissue).

The direct method has two advantages over the indirect method: first, it enables the use of long, thin needles; second, it allows the examination of tissues in which sound propagation velocities vary (fatty deposits).

When questions are raised in practice concerning the development of higher-contrast needles or the most favorable biopsy technique, several important physical principles should be considered. Because the direct method provides an inherently superior accuracy of localization, but this advantage is often not utilized because of poor needle visibility, an optimization of measuring procedures would appear to be indicated. Also, it is likely that further technical refinements of this method may be expected in the future.

Direct visualization of the needle shaft and tip is influenced by various factors. To understand these factors better, it is necessary first to consider how image contrast in a sonogram is obtained.

General Considerations on the Formation of Image Contrast in Sonograms

In echo-sonography acoustic reflectivity is the property of matter that is displayed on the monitor in the form of a brightness distribution pattern. Sound reflection from an object detail, such as an interface between two media, occurs

13

when the acoustic impedance $Z = \rho \cdot v$, where ρ is density and v is sound velocity, changes in the direction of the incident beam.

In the simple case of a flat boundary between two media that is at right angles to the beam axis and whose lateral dimension d is large in relation to the wavelength λ, the reflection coefficient R in Eq. (1) essentially determines the brightness of the echo [10, 90],

$$R = \frac{Z_2 - Z_1}{Z_2 + Z_1} \tag{1}$$

where Z_1 and Z_2 are the acoustic impedances of the two media. This is the case of specular reflection under normal incidence. If the reflector is tilted, the echo wave finally will miss the transducer (which is as a rule the same for transmitting and receiving), and the object will not be imaged. Under specular conditions thin membranes also reflect at the angle of glare, i.e., in accordance with the law of optical reflection, though with a relatively small reflection coefficient.

Another easily described boundary case is that of a particle which is very small in relation to the wavelength, i.e., $d < \lambda$. Here the nature of the interaction of the sound and target is the same as in the case described above, but the law of reflection no longer applies. This case is governed by the principles of a wave phenomenon known as scattering. Echo intensity in the presence of scattering is strongly influenced by a quantity called the scattering cross-section S. Besides Z_1 and Z_2, the scattering cross-section depends on the target diameter d and the wavelength λ as defined by the relation [90, 170]

$$S \sim \frac{d^3}{\lambda^2} \tag{2}$$

Tiny, isolated particles have a very broad or spherical scattering characteristic. Their shape and position have little influence on the brightness of the echo. They are always visible, given a sufficient impedance difference, because they always reflect some of the incident energy back to the transducer. On the other hand, even large objects may return no signal at all if they have smooth surfaces and do not reflect toward the transducer. This seems paradoxical when compared with diagnostic radiology and illustrates how different the two modalities are in their mechanisms of image generation.

In the case where $d \approx \lambda$, a complex echo pattern results, and the shape and position of the particles begin to have an effect on the scatter curve.

Human Tissue. By virtue of its cellular composition, human tissue is intricately structured and hence is a scatterer of sound. In the case of fine tissue structures and blood particles that cannot be resolved sonographically, we are dealing with very small scatterers that do not occur in isolation. Models that attempt to describe the scattering of sound from different human tissues are based on random distributions of particles whose acoustic impedances vary in a discontinuous manner [170]. Transitional cases (d ≈ λ) with broad scattering functions that are maximal at an angle of glare also occur frequently in tissues.

Only flat, macroscopic tissue structures (d > λ) reflect strongly marked specularly, though with a moderate reflectivity. Specular reflections occur at interfaces between organs and fluid-filled spaces, for example, and at the walls of the larger blood vessels. They are visualized by the usual scanners with high contrast, when the structures are normal to the interrogating beam.

Thus it will be appreciated that all possibilities for echo generation, including boundary cases, exist in human tissues, and that scattering predominates. With the exception of bone, air-tissue interfaces, and concretions, strong reflections do not occur in body tissues.

Biopsy Needle

With an artificial object such as a large, smooth, metallic foreign body, the situation is reversed: scattering is of minor importance compared with specular reflection at the interface between the quasi-fluid body tissue and the metal. A very strong echo-wave is produced owing to the marked impedance discontinuity that exists at the interface.

Needle Shaft. Because of its size (d > λ) and smooth surface, the *shaft of a needle* is considered to be a specular reflector. It yields a very bright image when interrogated with a normally incident beam. In an obliquely incident beam, it is rendered visible only by virtue of its „material flaws," i. e., scratches and roughness on the outer and inner surface of the needle or on the stylet, or the presence of small gas bubbles [67]. These irregularities are a source of weak scattered waves. In the water bath, a needle shaft appears as an irregular series of echoes of varying brightness when the contrast control of the instrument is suitably adjusted. Flaws of this type, however, are not echogenic enough to permit the consistent and reliable recognition of the shaft in tissue.

Artificial roughening of the needle shaft can markedly improve its sonographic visualization. Of course, limits are set to this roughening by the possibility of tissue traumatization.

In the Japanese fine needle (Hakko Shoji Tokyo), for example, the shaft is made visible by a series of very fine, irregularly spaced grooves on the outside of the shaft and on the stylet. Water bath experiments show that this microroughness promotes the formation of tiny air bubbles on the roughened surfaces, which influence the intensity of scattering. However, this needle does not appear to offer significant advantages for practical use (see also p. 33 ff). A regular surface profile, such as a spiral-shaped groove, has proved highly effective under experimental conditions. This feature was probably first incorporated into the amniocentesis needle of Jonatha [82]. When irradiated with ultrasound, these equidistant scatterers produce a grating effect that leads to constructive or

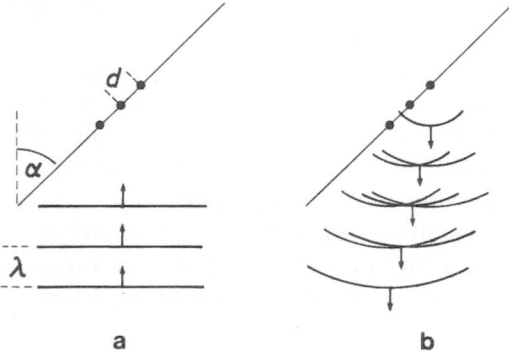

Fig. 8 a,b. Diffraction of a short wave train with three periods incident on a linear point grating. Three adjacent grating elements are considered. **a** α, angle of incidence; d grating constant; λ, wavelength; *black arrows*, direction of incident wave. **b** Backscattered waves, which interfere constructively in the direction of the transducer; see also Eq. (3) in text

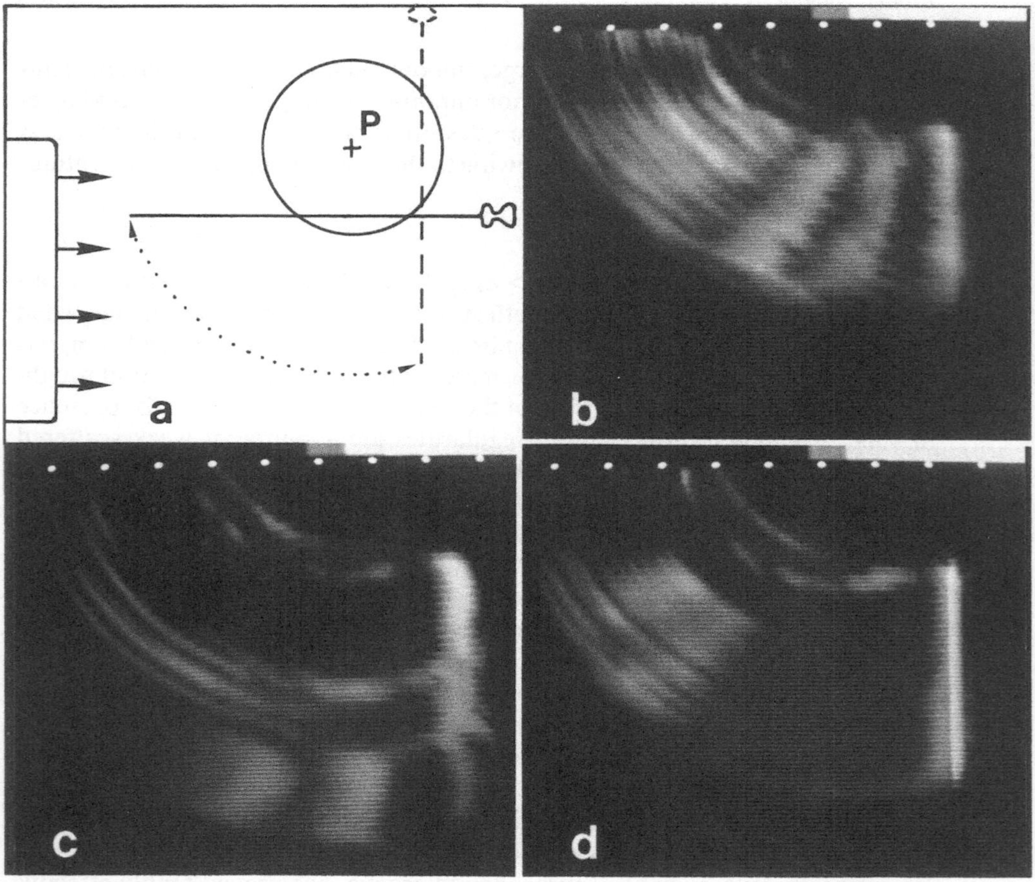

Fig. 9 a-d. Demonstration of the grating effect. **a** The needles were attached to a disk and rotated 90° in a water bath while a time exposure was made. Imaging device: B-scanner (Toshiba SAL 20 A). **b-d** Brightness diagrams of the Jonatha needle, the Nordenström needle, and the prepared fine needle

destructive interference of the scattered wave trains. In this way certain beam angles will cause scattered energy to be directed back toward the transducer, so that an image of the shaft is produced in an obliquely incident beam. Figure 8 a,b illustrates the pattern of wave interference that occurs in such a case. According to simplified theoretical assumptions, the sound amplitude A is related to the spacing d and angle of incidence α by the equation

$$A(d, \alpha) = \cos^2 \frac{2\pi \cdot d \cdot \cos\alpha}{\lambda} \tag{3}$$

Elsewhere, we have shown [30] that this brightening effect can also be achieved with fine needles having surface irregularities no larger than 0.02 mm. Figure 9 a-d shows an experiment that demonstrates the grating effect in three different needles. In this experiment the needles are rotated in the ultrasound field, and a photographic time exposure is made to show the brightness distribution for different angles of sound incidence. Figure 9 b shows that the Jonatha needle returns echoes over almost the entire range of angles, with conspicuous diffraction maxima and minima. These agree well with the formula given above. With the corkscrew-like stylet of the Nordenström needle, only two maxima are observed at incidence angles between 45° and 90°. The prepared fine needle also shows two maxima occurring between 0° and 45°. If a high-precision raster is used, it will not only increase the overall brightness of the needle, but will also (unlike irregular roughening) make the brightness appear uniform. Such an object is relatively conspicuous in tissue, where it is surrounded by irregularly distributed scatterers.

Needle Tip. In the smooth, unprepared needle, it is a fortunate circumstance that the *needle tip*, representing an abrupt discontinuity in the homogeneously reflecting shaft, is almost always visualized with ultrasound as a „material flaw." The notion of a needle tip producing an echo may seem curious at first, especially in cases of small angles of incidence. But the phenomenon is easily understood in terms of the laws of diffraction, and the basic principle has been known for many years. As early as 1802, Young observed in studies of light waves that the edge of a diffracting object appears bright when observed from the region of the geometric shadow. His theory of the „boundary wave," which arises from the edge of the object and illuminates the shadowed area, has proved correct and has been theoretically confirmed for the general case (Rubinowicz form of the Kirchhoff diffraction integral [14]). This means that the needle tip always scatters energy as a result of diffraction.

Explaining the needle tip echo in terms of a boundary wave is not inconsistent with the explanation of Goldberg and Ziskin [53], who, by analogy with sound propagation in tubes, ascribe a change of impedance to the sudden change in beam cross section at the end of the needle. However, the diffraction formalism allows a more general treatment of the problem in the case of both the tip and the shaft and, above all, provides an explanation for the wavelength-dependent phenomena that are observed.

To describe in more accurate terms the action of a needle tip in a wave field, we must take into account a variety of effects and conditions that may be summarized as follows:

1. On the one hand, the needle tip belongs to the class of objects with $d \approx \lambda$, which is not easy to deal with theoretically. On the other, the tip cannot be considered in isolation from the shaft.
2. A portion of the sound energy penetrates the needle, setting up a transverse wave and various associated waveforms that depend on the geometry of the needle and the wavelength λ. These influence the proportion of energy that is backscattered to the transducer.
3. Scattering alters the acoustic spectrum. The effects also depend on the filtering properties of the medium (water bath, tissue).
4. Needle tips vary greatly in their design, bevel, stylet, and other features.

In the present context, then, it is easier to approach these questions experimentally. Qualitative tests under waterbath conditions already reveal a marked dependence of echo intensity I on imaging geometry.

Experimental Comparison of Different Needle Types

A-scan Instrument. First we shall examine the case where the needle is coaxial with the ultrasound beam, i. e.,where the angle of incidence α is $0°$ or very small. Using a biopsy transducer with a central lumen and an A-scan instrument in conjunction with a water bath, it is easily shown how different needle types vary in their echogenicity and what effect a stylet has.

In the models tested, we noticed that the position of the stylet in the shaft can greatly influence the brightness of the needle tip echo, even when the tip of the stylet is relatively distant from the needle tip. If we define the dependence of the needle tip echo intensity I on the length x of the water-filled needle segment in front of the stylet as the „stylet function" (Fig. 10), we find that the needles can be divided into two groups based on the basis of the general shape of the curve I(x): one with a rising stylet function, as illustrated by the 0.7-mm Chiba needle, and one with a constant stylet function, as represented by the Jonatha needle, trocar needle, and Japanese fine needle. Another distinguishing feature is the oscillation of the curves, which varies markedly in its period and amplitude (see the diagrams in Table 1).

If the needle shaft is covered with a plastic sheath that leaves only a few millimeters of tip exposed, movements of the stylet under the sheath have no effect on tip brightness as long as air is present between the sheath and metal shaft. But if water enters this interspace, the typical oscillating function is again observed. The curves in the fourth and fifth lines of Table 1 show this clearly.

We may conclude from these effects that, in unsheathed metal needles, the incident wave and the wave scattered from the tip interact with the shaft and its contents as they travel along the needle. The oscillations in the stylet function

18

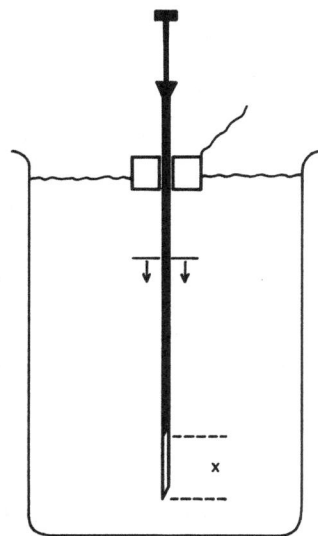

Fig. 10. Biopsy needle inserted into a water bath through the lumen of a monotransducer (x, water-filled segment of needle; *black arrows,* direction of transmitted sound pulse)

must be interpreted as interference. The periods of these oscillations point to the formation of wire waves that have a greater velocity than the water waves and are preferentially reflected at the tips of the needle and stylet.

Table 1 also shows the estimated intensities of the needle tip echoes and also of the shaft echoes for roughened needles. These estimates are intended to serve as a guideline. During the measurements the needles were allowed a lateral play of a few millimeters to simulate real biopsy conditions.

The brightest tip echoes were exhibited in the absence of a stylet by the Chiba-type needles (beveled) with outer diameters of 0.7–1.0 mm and our own experimental needle, which is a modification of the Chiba needle (Angiomed Co., D-7505 Ettlingen). The Japanese fine needle with irregular grooving is also of the Chiba type with respect to the shape of its tip, but it is a relatively poor acoustic reflector. Like the thinner Franzen needle, also a poor reflector, it differs from the other Chiba needles in the general shape of its stylet function.

In the Franzen needle, we also find that the tip of the thin, slightly curved cleaning wire within the shaft is far more echogenic than the needle tip itself. The increase of 4 dB on insertion of the stylet is attributed to the generation of wire waves. The same effect is observed when the cleaning wire is tested outside the needle shaft.

With regard to the larger-caliber needles listed in Table 1, it is noteworthy that a plastic sheath appears to inhibit the production of a needle tip echo even when the tip itself is left exposed. We also note that the tip of the trocar needle, which is designed for core biopsies, is not a very effective scatterer around 0° incidence.

Table 1. Comparative evaluation of needle echo characteristics in a water bath at about 0° beam incidence (biopsy tranducer with 13-mm aperture, 2.25 MHz, Toshiba; A-scope: USIP 11, Krautkramer; needle tip about 7 cm from transducer). The decibel scale was chosen such that the approximately equally intense echoes of the stylet-armed fine needles were at the 0 dB level

Needle type	Diameter [mm]	Stylet fully inserted Tip [dB]	Shaft [dB]	Without stylet Tip [dB]	Shaft [dB]	Stylet function, pattern of echo intensity curve (as function of x)	Remarks
Jonatha needle (spiral groove)	1,3	10	3	6	3		Amniocentesis, plastic coating, beveled
Trocar needle	1,2	0		0			Core biopsy, edged stylet tip
Reference needle	1,0	6		6			Rotationally symmetric tip rounded stylet tip
Plastic-sheathed needle with air interspace	1,6/1,0	−10		−6			Beveled
Plastic-sheathed needle with water coupling	1,6/1,0	−16		−4			Beveled
TSK Supra needles (Chiba type)	1,0 0,9 0,8			16 20 6			Disposable needles used without a stylet
Chiba needle	0,7	0		18			
Chiba needle (irreg. grooves)	0,7	0	−22	−4	−22		Measured without air bubbles (echo intensities greater when bubbles are present)
Our fine needle (spiral groove)	0,7	0	− 6	18	4		Measured without air bubbles (echo intensities greater when bubbles are present)
Franzen needle	0,6	0		−6			Normally used without stylet. Stylet effects were measured with a cleaning wire

20

The echogenicity of the roughened shaft or stylet on immersion of the dry needle in water is greatly enhanced by the presence of small air bubbles, as mentioned earlier. This effect subsides once the rough surfaces are completely wetted. In the present experiment, measurements were made with the surfaces wetted, since echo values in the presence of air bubbles are not well reproducible. Our fine needle with its echogenic groove raster proved superior to all the others tested in terms of shaft visibility in the A-mode display.

B-Scan Instrument. With B-scan instruments it is often possible to introduce the needle at an oblique angle relative to the ultrasound beam. The mechanical needle guide may be mounted on the side of the transducer, or it may be located at the center of a linear-array transducer. Thus we are considering the case where $\alpha > 0°$. We must also take into account the angle of rotation β about the long axis of the needle, as well as other parameters.

When the angle of incidence is continuously varied, strong fluctuations are observed in the brightness of the needle tip echo. This also occurs when the needle is rotated about its long axis, if the tip is not rotationally symmetric. Hjelmroth [69] recently presented examples of the function $I(\alpha)$ for various needle diameters and sound frequencies and showed how the tip signal also varied as a function of diameter and bevel. To the extent permitted by modulation of these curves through diffraction and interference effects, the following conclusions may be drawn:

1. When $\alpha = 0°$, larger-gauge needles yield a brighter image than smaller-gauge needles, as Goldberg and Ziskin [53] also demonstrated. This tendency is no longer evident when $\alpha > 0°$.
2. The function $I(\alpha)$ always attains a maximum at 90°, thus at the point where specular shaft reflection begins; the value of the function at that point is greater than the other maxima attained at different angles.
3. In arrangements with $\alpha = 0°$, a bevel of 0° is the most favorable. The signal becomes weaker as the bevel angle increases.
4. A higher frequency apparently leads to brighter needle tip echoes.

Of course, these rules apply only to the general shape of the function in question and usually prove imprecise when applied to specific cases. It would be helpful, therefore, to know the scattering characteristics of conventional needles more exactly.

With this in mind, we constructed the rotary apparatus shown in Fig. 11 and used it to test the backscatter characteristics of three different biopsy needles. Measurements were performed with an industrial A-scope that displayed echo intensity as a deflection on the y axis. The tip echo, which always appeared in the same place on the monitor screen, was isolated with a mask and photographed during one complete revolution with a open-shutter camera that rotated synchronously with the needle. With proper alignment of the rotational axes,

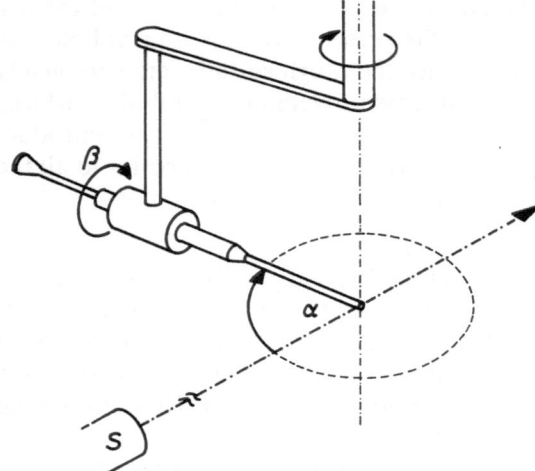

Fig. 11. Rotary apparatus for studying backscatter curves in a water bath. The ultrasound beam from probe S is kept trained on the needle tip as the angles α and β are varied

this setup produces a record of the angular dependence of I in the form of a polar diagram. As it revolved around its tip, the needle was also rotated about its long axis. If this latter rotation is performed at a relatively high number of revolutions per minute, a fine structure is superimposed on the backscatter function which gives useful information on the effect of variations of β.

The results of the experiment are shown in Fig. 12 a-c. The tests were run at frequencies of 2 and 5 MHz, and each characteristic was recorded at two contrast settings: first the maximum deflection at $\alpha=90°$ was brought to the full height of the scale (left image), and then the gain was increased by 20 dB (right image). Withdrawal of the stylet has only a slight effect on the contrast at 90° ($\lesssim 2$ dB). A comparison of the intensities at the two frequencies would be possible only if the probe and instrument sensitivities were precisely known or if a calibration standard were utilized. The range of $\alpha < 4°$ is excluded because of shadowing.

From a practical standpoint, it is interesting to note that:

1. Some of the backscatter curves exhibit additional strong maxima besides the one occurring at $\alpha=90°$.
2. The brightness of the needle tip at small angles of incidence can be markedly increased by dispensing with the stylet or by retracting it a few millimeters.
3. The scattering characteristic for small α is more favorable at the higher frequency than at the lower frequency (this effect is masked in the Chiba needle by strong secondary maxima).
4. Brightness is strongly dependent on rotational angle β when the tip is not rotationally symmetric;

22

2 MHz   5 MHz

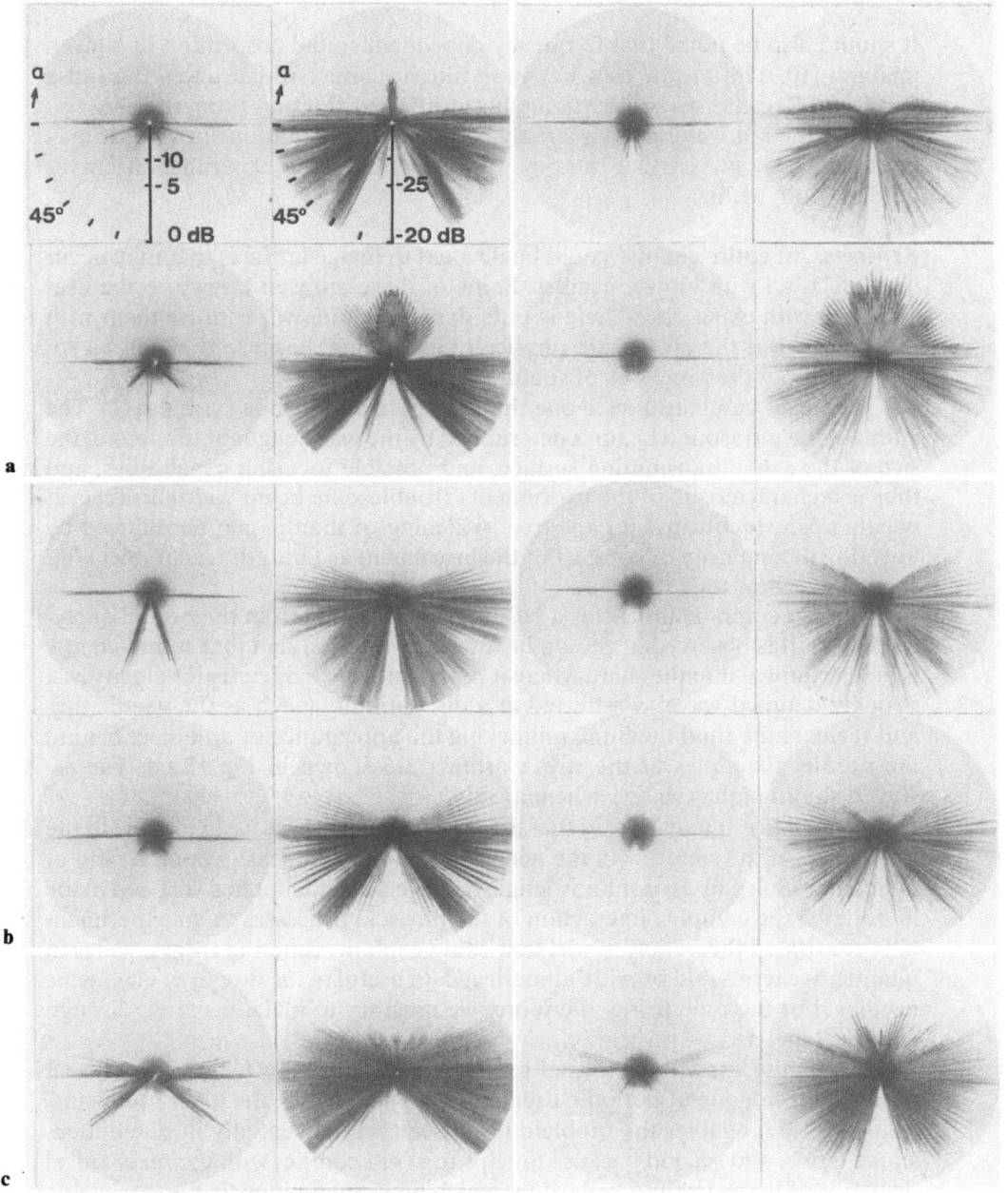

Fig. 12 a–c. Backscatter characteristics of three biopsy needles at 2 MHz and 5 MHz, recorded with the rotary apparatus in Fig. 11 and an industrial A-scan instrument (Krautkrämer USIP 11). The polar diagrams were recorded with the aid of a rotating camera (see text p. 21). The right image in each pair was made with the gain increased 20 dB over the left (α, angle of incidence). **a** Reference needle (1.0 mm, tip sharpened but unbeveled) with *(bottom)* and without a stylet *(top)*. **b** Chiba needle (0.7 mm, 65° bevel) with *(bottom)* and without a stylet *(top)*. **c** Trocar needle (1.2 mm) with stylet

5. The range of very small angles $\alpha > 0$ is always relatively unfavorable. Additional details are given in the legend to Fig. 12.

It should also be noted that frequency-dependent sound absorption in a given medium [10, 170] produces a low-pass filtering effect which alters the pulse spectrum. Because water and tissue have different filtering properties, the results obtained in water cannot strictly be applied to conditions in vivo. It may be assumed, however, that the gross effects seen in the experimental curves hold for both media.

Artifacts. An entire chapter could be devoted to image artifacts that may occur in association with biopsy needles. Some of these are well known to the user [67], and, with experience, there is little danger that he will confuse them with the needle. But the effects are physically interesting, because they tell us something about the processes of sound propagation.

The beam width artifact is one that occurs in all B-mode systems [12]. The width of the ultrasound beam is determined by the wavelength of the sound, the size of the active transmitting surface, and possible focusing capabilities, and thus is a characteristic of the instrument. Troublesome beam width artifacts at needle tips, which cause an apparent widening of the tip, can be reduced by lowering the intensity or contrast of the instrument as far as the anatomical image details allow this.

Another common artifact is a tail-like streak arising from the needle or stylet tip [67]. It is observed at certain beam angles and is a sign that sound energy is being coupled into the shaft, where it propagates at characteristic velocity as a strongly damped wave, is reflected at a discontinuity (such as the needle tip), and reenters the fluid medium, mimicking the appearance of an object behind the needle. Examples of the streak artifact are shown in Fig. 13 a,b. The assumed sound path is shown schematically.

In *summary,* it may be said that the fundamental effects associated with the interaction of the sound with the needle are known, not least from the field of material testing [90]. To our knowledge, however, no attempt has yet been made to describe the complex interaction of the physical processes in an experimentally confirmed theoretical model that could explain scattering from needles in quantitative terms and provide numerical data useful in the design of echogenic needles. For the time being, therefore, we must try to make progress through empirical means.

Among the known methods of increasing echo intensity [67], the somewhat neglected technique of periodic roughening appears to be the most promising, first because it enables the problem to be dealt with essentially in one-dimensional terms, and second because it helps to avoid conflict with the mechanical demands of tissue or fluid collection, which limit the options that are available for optimization of the needle tip.

To the user, we commend the advantages of a favorable geometry, i. e., optimum α and β angles and an optimum stylet position. The user should have

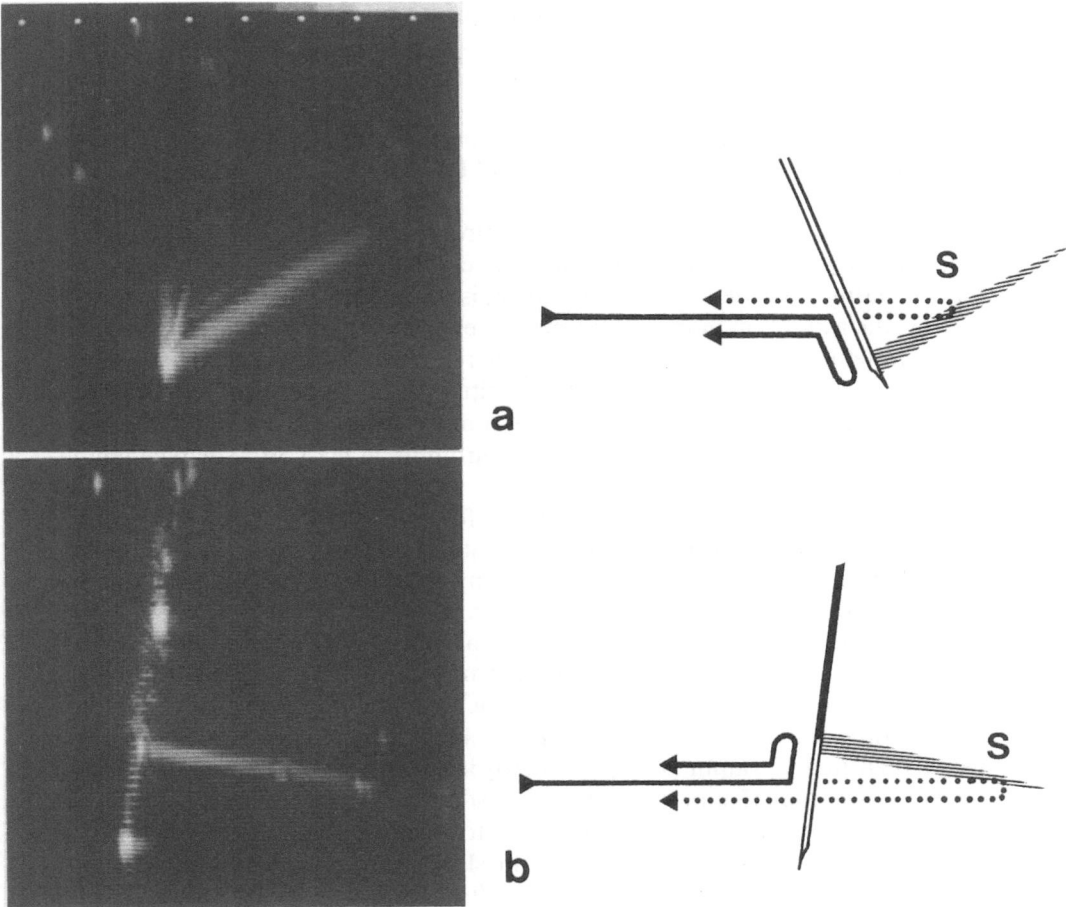

Fig. 13a,b. Streak artifacts in the B-mode image create the appearance of an object *(S)* behind the needle. The assumed path of the sound pulse is shown schematically *(arrow)*. **a** Three streaks prove the existence of three wave modes. The artifactual echoes are caused by reflection of the shaft wave at the tip. The needle is water-filled and is not visible. **b** Water-filled needle with stylet partially retracted. Here the reflection occurs at the tip of the stylet

some appreciation of the shape of the backscatter curve and of the stylet function $I(x)$ for the particular needle being used. If these quantities are unknown, a water bath test can be conducted to determine the most favorable parameters. Manufacturers of biopsy needles are urged to facilitate optimum use of their instruments by specifying the most favorable working parameters for each needle and offering appropriate types for the different examining conditions.

3 Procedure for Fine-Needle Aspiration Biopsy

3.1 Technique

First a standard real-time examination of the abdomen is performed. We recommend that both the upper abdomen and lower abdomen be scanned at one sitting.

If this routine examination discloses a circumscribed structural abnormality in a parenchymatous organ that is suggestive of a tumor, then the next step, after consulting with the referring physician, is to perform an ultrasound-guided fine-needle aspiration biopsy if this may be expected to provide additional useful information. Prior consultation with the referring physician, usually by telephone, is essential in order to identify any situation or condition that might contraindicate needle biopsy. Also, a biopsy should never be attempted unless the coagulation time is known (one-stage prothrombin at least 50%, platelet count at least $80\,000/mm^3$).

This brief communication is very useful for both sides. It provides the sonographer with important details about the patient that may not be stated on the referral sheet, and it helps the attending physician to choose additional diagnostic studies and manage his patient better.

For most aspiration biopsies we use a specially developed linear-array transducer with a central aperture. This transducer is not suitable for primary scans, because the central aperture (sight line) might interfere with the examination. At times this can make it difficult to relocate an inconspicuous lesion detected on primary examination, particularly if the frequency of the biopsy transducer is lower than that of the primary transducer. With experience, however, it is possible to compensate for this loss of information.

Once the lesion has been localized, the skin is antiseptically prepared as for surgery (see below), and the biopsy transducer is wrapped in a sterile plastic bag and applied to the skin directly over the lesion to be biopsied. The next step is to position the sight line of the transducer so that it intersects the target. When the operator has done this, he usually has his assistant steady the transducer in the selected position. It is possible for the operator to hold the transducer during the biopsy, but this has not proved practical. Now the fine needle with indwelling stylet is introduced through the central aperture of the transducer into the skin and subcutaneous fatty tissue (Fig. 14).

Local anesthesia of the skin, subcutis and peritoneum is unnecessary in most cases. The anesthesia is no less painful than the puncture itself, and it may lead to side effects. However, some patients are very sensitive to the pain of needle insertion and especially to puncture of the peritoneum, and so local anesthesia with 3–5 ml 1% lidocaine may be advised. This has two advantages: it accustoms the patient to the pain of the needle, and it makes it easier to reach smaller targets because the patient remains quieter. The disadvantage of local anesthesia is that the patient must be starved. Some patients complain of dizziness and nausea after the injection.

26

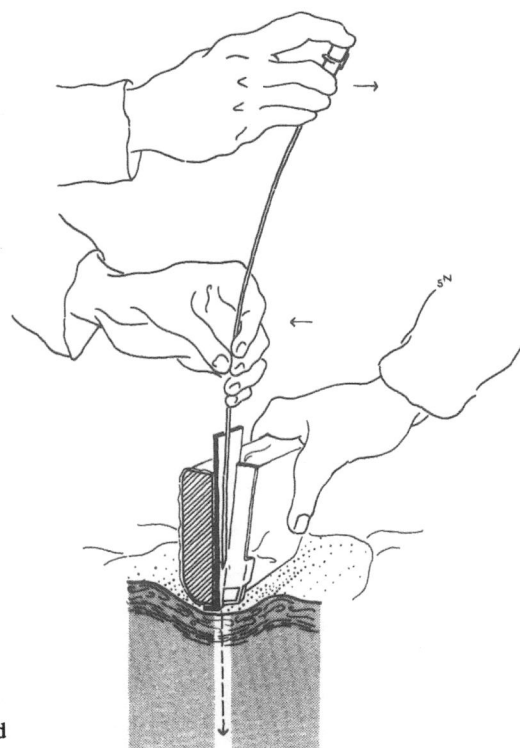

Fig. 14. Method of holding the elastic fine needle when introducing it through the transducer (cut away to show wedge-shaped aperture)

As soon as the biopsy needle has entered the skin, strict care must be taken that it does not stray from the tomographic plane of the transducer; otherwise it will not be visible. The plane of the scan is only about 1 mm wide. To ensure an accurate entry of the fine needle, one may either use a preformed wedge with a small guide tube (Fig. 15 b), or bow the needle slightly and brace it against the back surface of the open guide slot, as was done in the older version (Figs. 14 and 15). A small guide tube is particularly useful for beginners, as it ensures that the biopsy needle will leave the transducer at the correct location.

The wedge-shaped aperture of the transducer is open at the front to permit some maneuvering of the needle and transducer during the procedure. This also allows complete removal of the transducer, which is helpful in cases where the puncture is to be followed by the injection of contrast material for radiographic imaging (cyst, bile ducts, antegrade pyelography, direct visualization of pancreatic duct, etc.).

In contrast to the water bath (p. 41), where the needle tip is visible at a depth of only about 1 cm, the needle tip must reach a depth of about 1.4 cm in tissue before it can be visualized. An easy way to increase the brightness of the needle tip is by retracting the stylet a few millimeters (Fig. 15 a,b). The physical basis of this maneuver was explained in the preceding chapter.

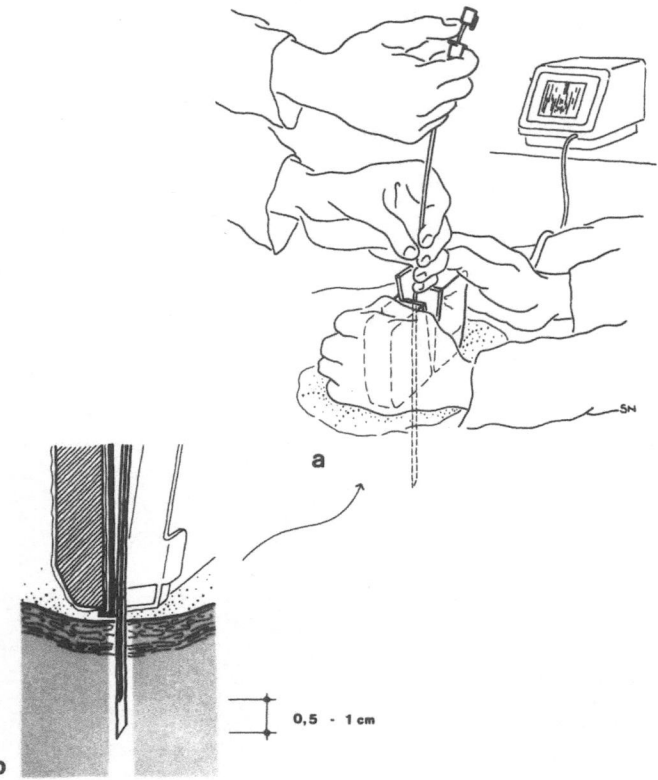

Fig. 15a, b. The stylet is retraced slightly to improve visualization of the needle tip

Given the small caliber of the needle, there is no need to fear that the tip will become clogged with unwanted material as it is pushed toward the biopsy site. Considerable suction with a 10-ml syringe is necessary in order to aspirate a significant amount of cellular material. Even when a fine needle is introduced without a stylet, a specimen can still be retrieved from deep within the body, though there will be some contamination with cells from the skin and intervening organs.

Individual Steps of the Aspiration Biopsy

For biopsies of the various organs, the needle is first introduced through the skin and into the subcutaneous fatty tissue. At this point there is time to prepare the patient for the somewhat painful passage of the needle through the peritoneum and organ capsule. First the patient is told to inhale and exhale deeply; the operator then thrusts the needle quickly through the peritoneum and organ capsule (e. g., of the liver), a distance of 2-3 cm.

When the needle tip has reached the desired location, the stylet is removed

28

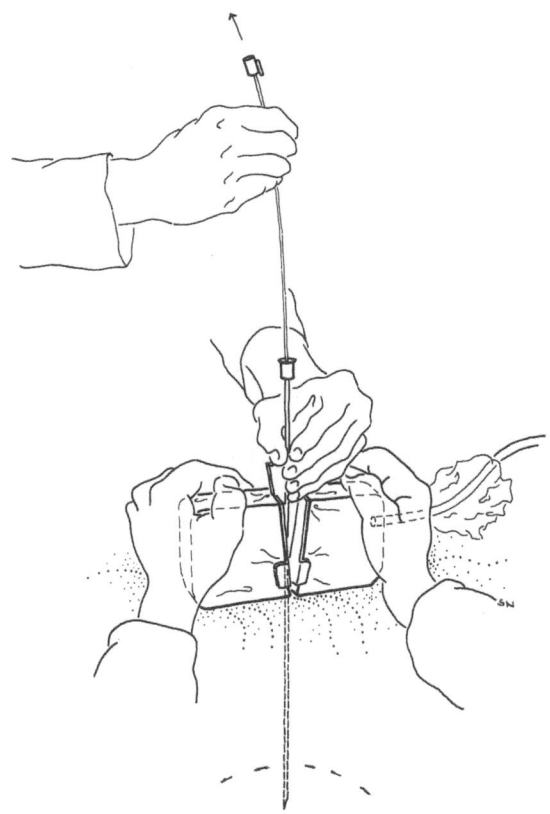

Fig. 16. When the needle tip has reached the area of interest, the stylet is completely removed

(Fig. 16) and a 10-ml plastic syringe with adaptor is connected to the hub to form an airtight seal (Fig. 17). Then the plunger of the syringe is moved upward with the thumb several times to create a vacuum of 1–5 ml that will aspirate the cellular material. As this is done, the needle and syringe are moved up and down a few millimeters in order to detach and aspirate a greater number of cells (Fig. 18). For some tumor consistencies this technique is necessary for a successful biopsy.

Auxiliary instruments may be used to facilitate movement of the plunger and increase the suction. They have two disadvantages, however: preparations for the procedure are more time-consuming, and it is more difficult to control the amount of suction applied. Because aseptic technique is used, it is also necessary to sterilize these parts prior to use.

Often it is necessary to biopsy well-perfused organ regions and tumors, in which case only a small amount of suction applied through a needle inserted into the periphery of the target will yield a good specimen. Excessive suction will aspirate mainly blood, from which tumor cells are almost impossible to recover.

As he gains experience with fine-needle biopsies, the operator will learn how to assess the quality of a focal lesion and vary his technique accordingly.

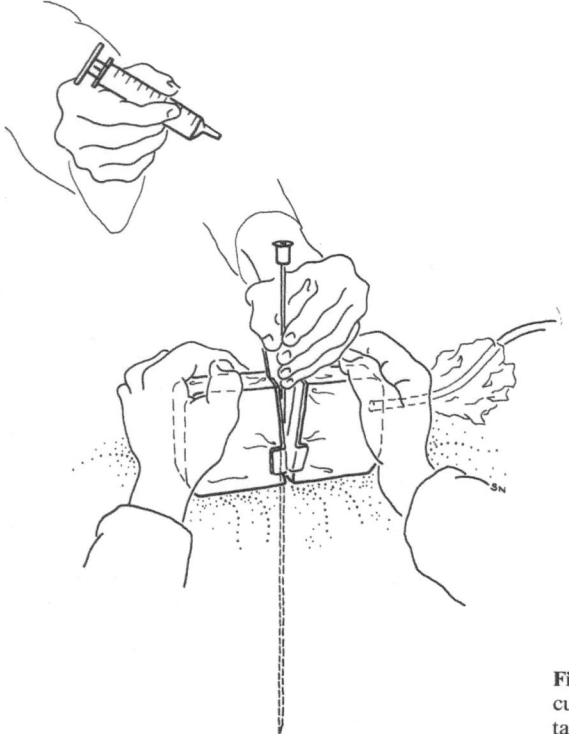

Fig. 17. The position of the needle is secured, and a 10-ml plastic syringe is attached for the aspiration

Thus he will find that a relatively forceful aspiration is needed to collect cells from a bowel tumor, while a hepatic hemangioma requires only a small amount of suction combined with a short, jabbing ("harpoon-like") movement of the needle into the lesion.

Before the needle is withdrawn, the plunger is allowed to return slowly to its original position (Fig. 19). Otherwise the carefully collected cellular material might pass into the syringe, from which it cannot be recovered quickly enough to spread onto a glass slide.

After the needle is withdrawn, pressure is applied as needed to control superficial bleeding, and the site is dressed with a simple adhesive strip. Afterward we observe the patient for up to 30 min. If pain persists beyond that point (which we have found to be very unusual), we extend the observation period and perform another ultrasound scan so that significant complications will not be overlooked. To date we have found no sonographic evidence of hemorrhage following aspiration biopsies with the Chiba needle.

Following core biopsies, closer observation over a longer period is advised, although the procedure may be done on an outpatient basis in selected cases.

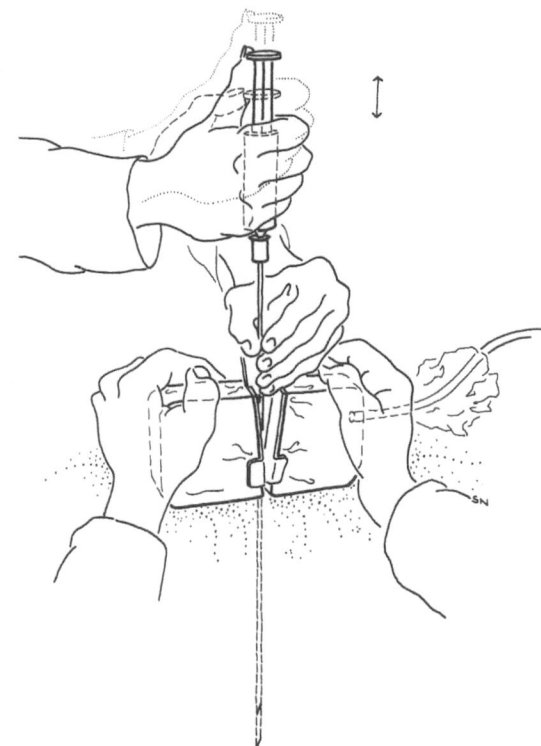

Fig. 18. The plunger of the syringe is moved upward while the needle is moved up and down slightly within the lesion

3.2 Technical Aspects

When performing fine-needle aspiration biopsies for the collection of material for cytologic or bacteriologic evaluation, we use a highly elastic, stylet-armed, Chiba-type needle [166] (Angiomed, D-7505 Ettlingen) with an outer diameter of 0.7 mm. Both needle and stylet are beveled (Fig. 20). The needle tip appears in sonograms as a bright point of light, even when the needle is introduced through the central aperture of our linear-array transducer and thus is directed parallel to the sound beam.

There are two main advantages of using a stylet with this needle:

1. Introduction of the needle is easier and less painful. Bending of the needle is avoided.
2. The needle is not contaminated by material traversed on the way to the biopsy site. Once the target is reached, the stylet is removed, freeing the lumen of the needle for the reception of tissue.

Because localization of the needle tip is made easier by retracting the stylet, especially if the tip has strayed from the plane of the scan, this maneuver is highly recommended. The stylet may be withdrawn several millimeters without clogging the tip.

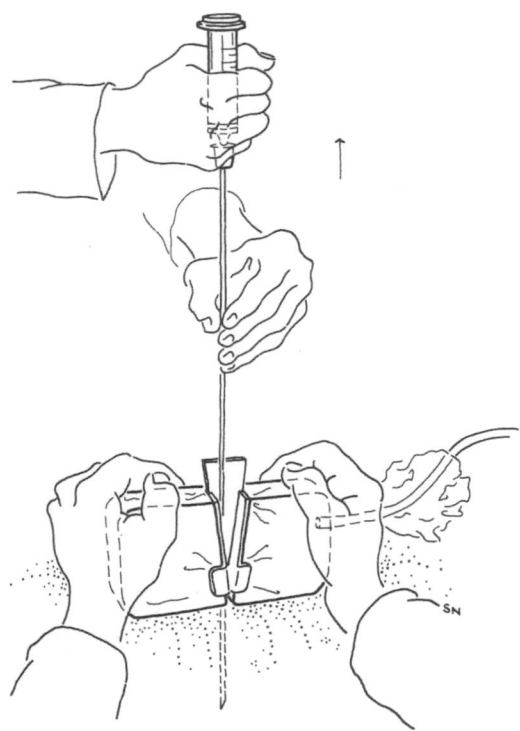

Fig. 19. The biopsy needle is withdrawn after first letting the plunger return to its original position

3.3 Methods of Improving Needle Tip Visibility

The visibility of the needle tip within the body is influenced by certain physical parameters (see p. 12ff.) and by factors relating to the depth of needle insertion and the characteristics of the area to be biopsied. Various phenomena associated with reflection of the ultrasound beam play a role. It is known that abrupt changes of acoustic impedance cause a partial or complete reflection of incident sound. However, as in optics, only a small fraction of the emitted energy is returned at normal incidence to the receiver.

Beam width artifacts are a common occurrence with strong reflectors such as needle tips. They are typically observed in hypoechoic areas, in the water bath, and in larger cysts [12]. Since ultrasound beam width increases with depth, the apparent widening of the needle tip echo can become troublesome at depths beyond 12–15 cm. Fortunately, potential biopsy sites rarely occur at this depth. (The origin of beam width artifacts has not been established with certainty, and they must relate in some fashion to side lobes, or energy maxima occurring outside the center of the main beam [107, 165].)

Except at extreme depths, beam width artifacts do not seriously interfere with ultrasound-guided biopsies, though at times it may be difficult to puncture a minimally dilated bile duct in the liver because of apparent tip widening.

32

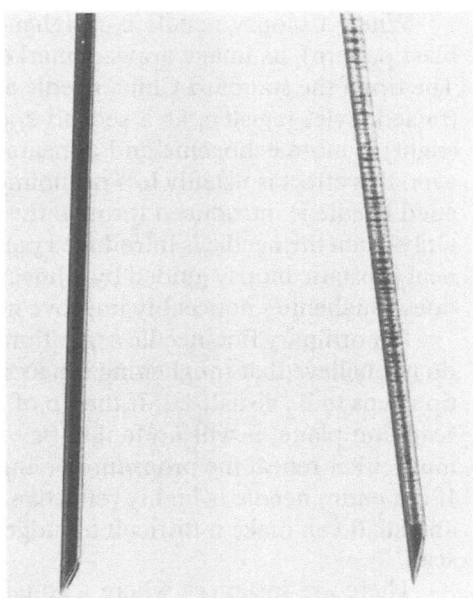

Fig. 20. Chiba needles: *left*, with smooth surface; *right*, with roughened surface

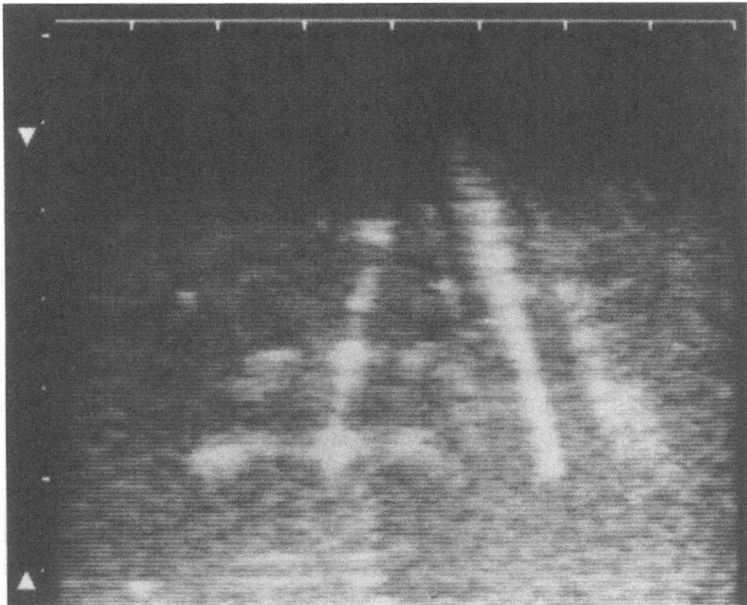

Fig. 21. Needles from Fig. 20 in a water bath. *Left*, the standard Chiba needle. The tip of the needle and of the retracted stylet are visible as bright points of light. *Right*, Chiba needle with roughened surface. The entire roughened shaft is clearly visible but contrasts poorly with the tip

33

When a biopsy needle is roughened externally (Fig. 20; annular or sandblast pattern), its image appears markedly different in the water bath (Fig. 21). The tip of the standard Chiba needle appears very bright, and the tip of the retracted stylet registers as a second spot of light (left). The roughened needle (right) is more echogenic and appears wider than the untreated needle. However, this effect is usually less pronounced in tissue, especially when the roughened needle is introduced through the central aperture of a biopsy transducer. Only when the needle is introduced parallel to a linear transducer (e. g., for perineal prostatic biopsy guided by a linear-array transducer inserted transrectally) does roughening noticeably improve needle visualization.

For ordinary fine-needle aspiration biopsies under ultrasound guidance, we do not believe that roughening is necessarily advantageous, for only the needle tip needs to be visualized. If the tip of a highly elastic needle deviates from the scanning plane, it will no longer be visible on the monitor, and the operator must either repeat the procedure or angle the transducer until the tip is located. If the entire needle is highly reflective, the absence of contrast between the tip and shaft can make it difficult to judge whether the tip has left the plane of the scan.

There are instances where a roughened needle offers certain advantages, such as in perineal biopsies performed under the guidance of a transrectal probe (prostate). Here the roughened needle will contrast more sharply with surrounding echogenic tissues than would a smooth Chiba needle. This also applies to biopsies of strongly fibrotic tissue, such as pleural thickenings and certain intestinal tumors.

3.4 Difficult Biopsy Sites

In principle, very superficial structures such as the breast and thyroid are more difficult to biopsy with the apertured linear-array transducer, because the needle tip is clearly visible only at a depth of about 10 mm, even under optimum conditions. (The exact depth depends on the angle between the tip bevel and the scanning plane and between the needle axis and crystal plane of the transducer.)

Lesions that require an intercostal route of approach, such as cranially situated hepatic tumors and intrathoracic masses (e. g., where biopsy is carried out to differentiate between pleural thickening and pleural tumor), are occasionally very difficult to biopsy under sonographic guidance. Apparently, much of the energy scattered from the needle tip is caught and reflected by the ribs, and the waves returned to the transducer are too weak to register on the monitor. It can be helpful in such cases to observe closely the traversed tissue layers, which will be displaced slightly as the needle tip is pushed forward.

Even in fibrotic tissue that is highly echogenic and reflects more energy than it transmits, the needle tip echo is occasionally lost because such structures greatly attenuate energy scattered from the needle tip, making it difficult or impossible to identify in the sonogram. Thus we have sometimes had difficulty locating the needle tip in a thickened pleura when attempting to differentiate a pleural tumor from a simple induration (e. g., secondary to tuberculosis) by means of aspiration cytology.

To help keep the atraumatic but highly elastic fine needle within the boundaries of the millimeter-wide image plane, we hold the transducer parallel to the longitudinal axis of the body whenever possible. When a voluntary or even involuntary respiration (e. g., on puncture of the peritoneum) causes displacement of the intraperitoneal organs or suspected tumor, the needle tip will tend to stay in the image plane and remain visible despite respiratory movements. This is important even in biopsies of retroperitoneal organs such as the pancreas, for these organs, too, may be displaced by respiration.

If the transducer cannot be oriented longitudinally over the biopsy site, it is often helpful to hold it in a nonstandard position that will still permit visualization of the lesion and proper alignment of the sight line. However, the biopsy will be more difficult and will require that the patient suspend respiration while the needle is advanced. Once the needle tip has passed 1–2 cm through the capsule of the target organ or has reached the biopsy site, we let the patient resume shallow respiration. This avoids possible laceration of the organ capsule, which may result in profuse hemorrhage requiring emergency intervention.

Some patients are incapable of breath-holding (resting dyspnea, uncooperativeness, etc.). If the needle tip echo is lost in such a situation, it can usually be relocated by angling the transducer slightly.

A special problem relates to the performance of biopsies in children. If the child is old enough and responsive to instructions, aspiration biopsy can usually be done under general sedation without the need for deeper anesthesia. The youngest of our biopsy patients, who required neither local nor general anesthesia, was just 3 years old (infected pulmonary cysts). In infants and small children, it is generally wise to administer a short-acting general anesthetic, as this will lower the risk of the procedure and improve the diagnostic yield.

If the biopsy needle cannot be definitively identified in the tissue, it is best to withdraw it completely, check it for bending and, if it is straight, reintroduce it. Rarely we have had to make up to five attempts at one sitting in order to obtain a diagnostic specimen (e. g., transcaval biopsy of a very small adrenal metastasis more than 12 cm deep). If the patient's prothrombin time and platelet count are satisfactory, we consider it reasonable to make up to five biopsy attempts in exceptional cases (see Sect. 3.1).

Of course, the risk of the biopsy depends on the body region involved, the intervening organs, and especially on the caliber of the biopsy needle. The use of core needles for the collection of histologic specimens places fundamentally different demands on the operator.

When larger needles like the Tru-Cut needle are used to obtain tissue for histologic study, adequate local anesthesia is mandatory. In addition, a scalpel must be used to make a 5-mm stab incision in the skin, into which the relatively blunt needle is superficially introduced. When the tip of the needle is within the subcutaneous tissue, the transducer is placed over the entry site, the needle fitting into its open, V-shaped central aperture in such a way that the needle shaft is on the image plane of the transducer. Care is taken to maintain firm contact between needle and transducer throughout the procedure. A deviation of the needle axis from the image plane by only 1 mm is sufficient to prevent sonographic visualization of the needle.

When a core biopsy is performed, it is imperative that the biopsy be taken with breathing suspended, for core needles are more rigid than fine aspiration needles, and there is a greater danger of seriously lacerating the tissue capsule, especially in the presence of inflammatory disease or certain types of neoplasm.

Under continuous sonographic vision, the operator can follow the needle tip precisely and, in the case of renal biopsy, direct it into the perirenal fatty tissue just outside the capsule. The risk of hemorrhage is increased only when the capsule is reached.

The design of the Tru-Cut needle allows for a very rapid excision of tissue. Cutting-edge needles, on the other hand, are considerably thinner and more flexible, the small-caliber types being highly elastic, and they may therefore remain within the organ for a brief moment during shallow respiration. This can be advantageous in uncooperative patients.

Cutting-edge needles also allow multiple core biopsies to be taken at a single sitting, for the thinner needles pose a smaller risk of primary hemorrhage. The somewhat greater effort involved in obtaining the specimen and recovering it for pathohistologic study is more than justified by the reduced risk to the patient.

The introduction of small catheters and drainage tubes into body cavities is performed in analogous fashion under sonographic guidance (see below). However, the patient should be premedicated with a sedative (5–10 mg diazepam) because the procedure is somewhat more painful than a needle biopsy. Alternatively, a half ampule of meperidine may be administered 30 min before the procedure.

If the structure to be punctured is well dilated or distended by pressure (marked hydronephrosis, suprapubic drainage of the urinary bladder, aspiration of ascitic fluid, abscess drainage, etc.), and it is reasonable to expect that the procedure will go quickly and smoothly, premedication may be adjusted accordingly. Special guidelines apply to punctures of the biliary tract.

3.5 Local Anesthesia and General Preparations

Years of experience have shown that local anesthesia is generally unnecessary for fine-needle aspiration biopsies. It is recommended only in some cases to accustom the patient to the pain of the needle insertion and in very sensitive patients to facilitate puncture of the peritoneum. Certainly, the more liberal use of local anesthesia is advised if the operator has had limited experience with the technique and if multiple biopsies are to be taken in succession.

Generally, this is all the preparation needed for a fine-needle aspiration biopsy. As a local anesthetic, we use 3-10 ml 1% lidocaine. We have not observed any anaphylactoid side effects with this agent. Nausea and dizziness have occasionally been reported after the biopsy, mainly by older patients, and so it is a good precaution to starve the patient before administering an anesthetic, and indeed before performing percutaneous biopsies in general.

In our experience, side effects from the procedure are referrable more to the local anesthesia than to the biopsy itself, although it has been shown that intra-abdominal biopsies can injure branches of the autonomic nervous system, leading to complications [164].

Even with a cutting-edge needle, local anesthesia may not be absolutely necessary, depending on the needle caliber, although individual pain sensitivity is an important factor in that decision. While the thinnest cutting-edge needle has the same outer diameter (0.8 mm) as the conventional fine needle and is introduced in an analogous manner, we generally administer a local anesthetic when using the larger cutting-edge needles (outer diameter 1.15 mm). Preliminary skin incision is not required for any of the cutting-edge needles.

We attach much importance to sound psychological guidance of the patient, who will certainly be somewhat apprehensive about the procedure, possibly because of a negative experience with other, more painful examinations in the past. If the patient is told that the procedure is somewhat painful but that the pain lasts only a few seconds, he will be able to tolerate it better. Generally, pain is experienced only during movement of the needle through the skin, peritoneum, and occasionally the organ capsule. Complete withdrawal of the needle and its reinsertion through the skin elicit more pain than up-and-down movements of the needle tip within the organ. Nevertheless, if the fine-needle tip is lost from the monitor screen and cannot be located by angling the transducer, it is still best to remove the needle and start the procedure again.

4 Standard Biopsy Needles for Cytology, Histology, and Bacteriology

The most commonly used biopsy needles (Fig. 22) may be categorized according to the type of tissue they obtain (material for cytologic or histologic evaluation) and thus their mode of tissue collection, or they may be distinguished by their ability to be localized with ultrasound. The more traumatizing biopsy needles (Fig. 23) have been superseded by finer instruments such as the cutting-edge needle and, in neoplastic conditions, fine needles for aspiration cytology. Moreover, these small-caliber needles are more readily identified sonographically within the body than the large-caliber needles of the past generation.

The Chiba-type (or Franzen-type) fine needle, the largest-caliber cutting-edge needle, and the still larger Tru-Cut needle are compared in Fig. 24. Despite the considerably larger outer diameter of the Tru-Cut needle, the amount of tissue retrieved is only slightly greater than that collected with the cutting-edge

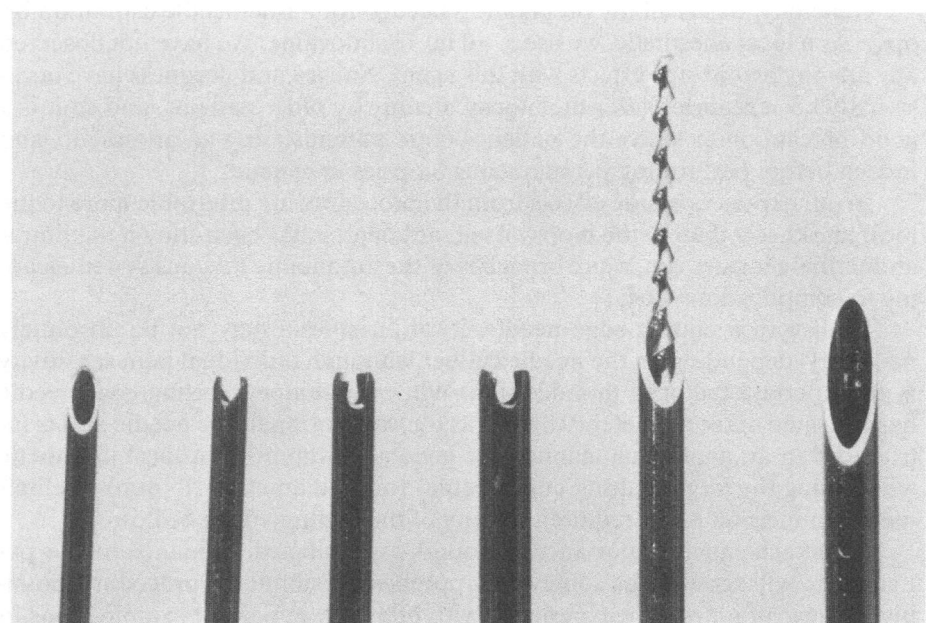

Fig. 22. *Far left,* Chiba needle; *2nd-4th from left,* Zurich cutting-edge needles; *far right,* Rotex needle. All the needles are shown in their working positions, as they would appear at the biopsy site

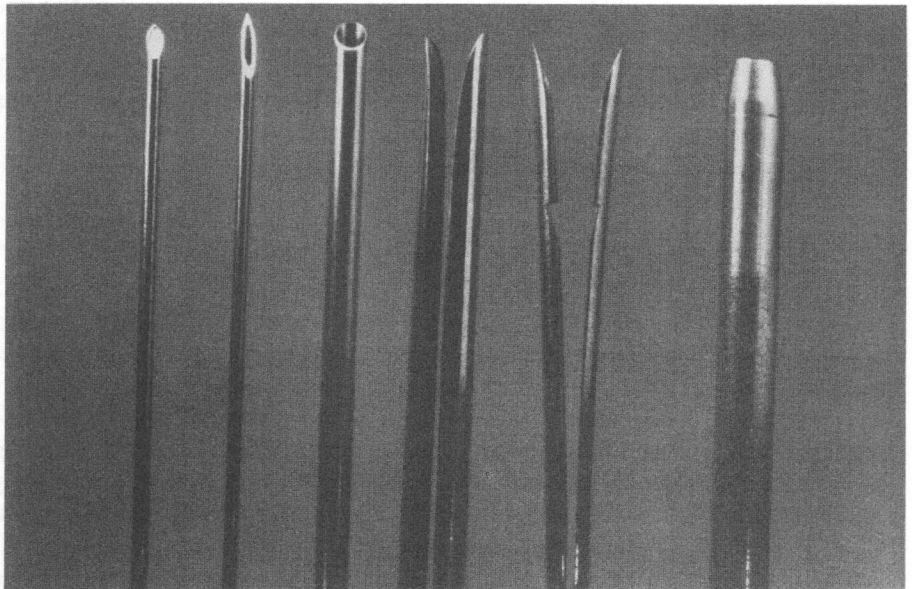

Fig. 23. Biopsy needles for obtaining cytologic and histologic specimens. *Left to right,* Chiba needle (for comparison), Franzen needle, Menghini needle, Silverman I and II split needles, trephine biopsy needle (of Hollinger)

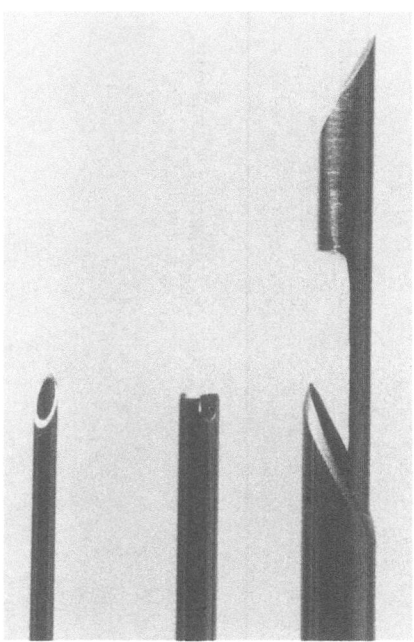

Fig. 24. Comparison of biopsy needles in the "working position." *Left,* Chiba needle (Angiomed). *Center,* largest-caliber cutting-edge needle (1.15 mm diameter). *Right,* Tru-Cut needle (for photographic reasons only partially opened). The wide end-piece of the obturator accounts for the necessarily large diameter of the needle and the relatively small tissue yield

needles. The latter usually provide considerably more tissue along the longitudinal axis of the needle (see Part C, Chap. 5, Fig. 52 a,b). Also, it is easier to justify multiple biopsies at one sitting with these needles than with a larger-caliber instrument.

For more precise evaluation of their sonographic qualities, these needles were tested using a linear-array biopsy transducer with a central aperture (Toshiba, Japan). First model tests were conducted in a water bath. To evaluate the brightest possible tip echo in a fine needle, for example, the tips were modified and their bevel angles varied. If a tip returned the brightest echo in the water bath, the same needle was also highly visible within the body, as expected. That needle then served as a pattern for the serial production of similar needles. The dimensions of different fine needles are very similar (Table 2). The three fine needles (Chiba type) compared by us are shown in Fig. 25.

Other needle types were tested in a similar fashion for the purpose of perfecting commercially available needles for use in ultrasound-guided biopsies.

According to Hjelmroth [69], the visibility of a needle tip in a sonogram depends on the material within the needle, the bevel of the tip, and the needle caliber. Our findings in this area are discussed in Part B, Chap. 2 and need not be repeated here in detail. We note, however, that when our biopsy technique is used, smaller-caliber, beveled needles are more visible during initial insertion than are larger-caliber needles and drainage tubes. Particularly strong echoes are returned by unbeveled stylets and from the vacuum at the needle tip.

Table 2. Characteristics of various biopsy needles

	Disposable needle	Reusable needle	Tip visibility	Tip bevel (degrees)	Diameter (mm) Outer/inner	Material for cytology or bacteriology	Histology	Therapeutic applications
Chiba needles:								
Angiomed	x		+ + +	24/23	0,68/0,43	x		Aspiration of small cysts, hematomas, etc.
Cook	x		+ +	23	0,71/0,45	x		
Unimed		x	+ +	24	0,71/0,45	x		
Cutting-edge needles:								
I	x		+ +	38	0,78/0,54	x	x	
II	x		+ +	41	0,93/0,68		x[a]	
III	x		+	48	1,15/0,90		x	
Follicular aspiration needle	x		+ +	17	1,19/0,83	Fluid with oocytes		Abscess drainage (liquid), aspiration of larger cysts
Rotex II	x		(+)	23	1,00/0,55/0,52	x		
Tru-cut	x		+/−	25	2,11/1,60		x	
Silverman			+/−	–	1,90–1,58		x	
Franzén			+ +	13	1,00/0,60	x		
Menghini			(+)	48	1,40		x	

−, none; +, fair; + +, good; + + +, excellent
[a] Depends on tissue composition

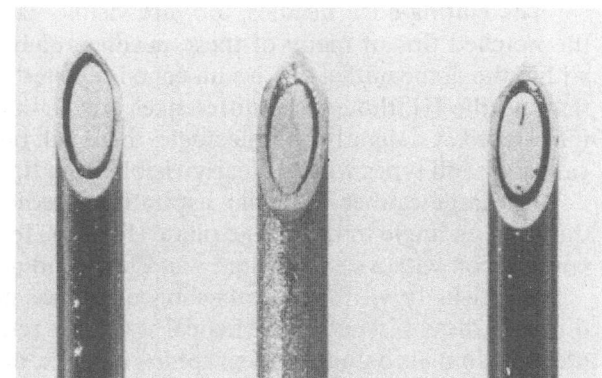

Fig. 25. Three different Chiba-type fine needles. *Left,* Angiomed (D-7505 Ettlingen). *Center,* Unimed (CH-1002 Lausanne). *Right,* Cook-Europa, (DK-Copenhagen)

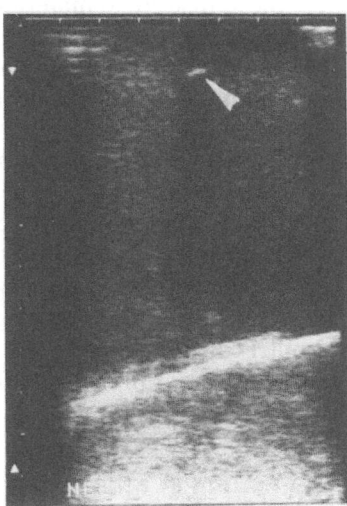

Fig. 26. The tip of the Chiba needle *(arrow)* is just visible at a depth of 1.2 cm (water bath)

The characteristics of the various biopsy needles are listed in Table 2. In view of the generally weaker tip echoes of larger-gauge needles, it is recommended that these needles be introduced through the transducer at a slightly oblique angle (see Fig. 60). A vertical insertion is more appropriate for fine-gauge needles. The heading "Tip visibility" relates exclusively to the use of a transducer with a central aperture.

The standard fine needles all have similar needle tip visibilities, although the original modified needles (Angiomed, D-7505 Ettlingen) exhibit a particularly strong tip echo, especially when the stylet is retracted slightly. Reusable needles (e.g., type 2R2 of Unimed, Lausanne) are disadvantageous because they must be thoroughly cleaned before use (time-consuming) and because they are gradually dulled with use. On the other hand, they are manufactured with very high precision and cause minimal artifactual echoes.

41

The cutting-edge needles, too, are visible when introduced vertically, but the notched tips of many of these needles require that the needle be rotated within the tissue until a maximum echo is elicited. Needles I and II are brighter than needle III, though the differences are slight. If the cutting-edge needle is introduced at a slightly oblique angle, there will be no difficulty whatever in localizing it; all types will be clearly visible from tip to shaft.

The large-caliber follicular aspiration needle is visible only when introduced at an angle to the image plane (Fig. 60). To date we have used it only in conjunction with a sector scanner and have had good results.

Surprisingly, we found that echogenicity was poorest with the Rotex II needle, regardless of whether the helical stylet was retracted or not. Today this needle is seldom used under sonographic guidance, and its most frequent use is for lung biopsies done under fluoroscopic control, as recommended by its designer. Because the cutting-edge needles are superior to the Rotex needle and collect more histologic material with the same or even less traumatization of tissues, we give preference to the cutting-edge types.

The Tru-Cut needle, which we used quite often until a few years ago, is difficult to image sonographically with sufficient clarity to localize its tip in tissue. Moreover, this needle is particularly traumatizing [130] and often causes considerable pain despite anesthesia (see also p. 98).

Accurate guidance of the needle in the tomographic plane of the transducer is of fundamental importance in ultrasound-guided biopsies. Only in this way can one be certain of visualizing the biopsy needle throughout the procedure. When a transducer with a central aperture is used, the needle cannot be followed until its tip has traversed the skin and subcutaneous tissue to a depth of about 1 cm (Fig. 26; see also Fig. 21). Thus superficial abnormalities of the thyroid, for example, can be difficult to biopsy under sonographic guidance.

C. Results

1 General

1.1 Indications and Methods of Specimen Collection for Cytologic, Bacteriologic, and Histologic Examination

It is imperative that histologic or at least cytologic proof of disease be obtained in cases where interventional therapy is indicated, such as the chemotherapy of a neoplastic process, and primary surgical treatment is not contemplated. When resective surgery is an option, a knowledge of the nature of the lesion will influence the planning of the operation or the decision to withhold surgery if the prognosis is poor. Owing to advances in instrumentation and the development of cytologic methods that usually allow a definitive diagnosis to be made from the analysis of a few cells or groups of cells, it is possible in many cases to establish the nature of a space-occupying lesion by fine-needle aspiration cytology.

A great many methods have been developed for obtaining cytologic or histologic material. They may be classified according to the type of guidance or instrumentation used (see also Table 3).

Table 3. Comparison of biopsy methods

Method	Purpose	Needle type	Risk[a]
Aspiration biopsy	Evaluation of tumors and abscesses, analysis of body fluids (cyst, pleural effusion, ascites, etc.)	Chiba and other fine needles (0.7–1 mm)	Low
Core biopsy, cutting biopsy	Evaluation of generalized renal or hepatic parenchymal disease, renal transplant, tumor diagnosis	Cutting-edge needle, Tru-Cut, Menghini, Silverman, etc.	Low Higher (bleeding, seeding of tumor cells)
Surgical drill biopsy[b]	Evaluation of generalized renal parenchymal disease (transplant rejection!), breast nodules, etc.	Trephine needle of Hollinger	Low, because performed under direct vision (usually intraoperative except in breast)

[a] Assuming safety controls are maintained (see p. 26)
[b] Guided not by ultrasound or computed tomography, but by palpation or direct vision

Methods of Obtaining Tissue Samples

1. Biopsy guided by palpation
   (e.g., breast, thyroid)
2. Laparoscopic biopsy under direct vision
   (e.g., tumor of pancreatic head, certain lower abdominal tumors)
3. Biopsy under conventional fluoroscopic control
   (e.g., lung biopsy, lymph node biopsy after lymphography, bone biopsy)
4. Ultrasound-guided biopsy
   a) Static scan
   b) Real-time scan:
      Sector scanner
      Linear scanner with central aperture
5. Computed-tomography-guided biopsy.

In the chapters that follow we shall describe a percutaneous biopsy method that has proved successful in various organs and in a large series of patients at our center. While this method makes no claim to exclusivity, it nevertheless enables a relatively rapid and accurate diagnosis to be obtained. Because pathologic examination is the most foolproof way to establish the identity of a suspicious lesion, it should be used to make the diagnosis. Also, the costs of the biopsy and laboratory analysis are fairly well standardized and considerably lower than for any other invasive procedure, since no costs are incurred by surgery or postoperative care. It is expected that this method will undergo further improvements and refinements with the passage of time (automation of specimen collection, simplification of laboratory processing, better documentation). Enthusiastic predictions of the diagnostic capabilities of nuclear magnetic resonance imaging, which allows tissue analysis by spectroscopic means, require further scrutiny. Nuclear magnetic resonance is a very costly technique and is appropriate only for a select group of patients.

1.2 Assessment of Diagnostic Accuracy

From 1978 to 1984, more than 3000 patients underwent percutaneous needle biopsies at our center under the guidance of real-time ultrasound or computed tomography. In 1802 of these patients we were able to compare the sonographic or computed tomographic diagnosis with the cytologic, histologic, or bacteriologic findings and with the final diagnosis. The latter was confirmed by surgery, autopsy, other diagnostic procedures (e.g., laparoscopy), or in some cases by clinical follow-up (e.g., clinical evidence of pancreatic cancer with suspicious computed tomographic scan but negative cytologic findings and several years' survival without clinical progression). The results are reported in a separate paper [17].

We were unable to evaluate the biopsy results in a larger population with regard to errors of methodology, because the further course of the disease could not be established with accuracy. Also, we were unable to determine the exact cause of death in many patients referred from abroad who died intercurrently. In principle it would seem reasonable to include malignant tumors diagnosed by biopsy in our statistics, but because false-positive diagnoses of malignancy are virtually nonexistent in cytology, inclusion of these cases would distort the accuracy rates.

Because our review includes patients from the early period of ultrasound-guided biopsy as well as more recent cases examined after the technique was improved, the results presented here represent a statistical mean and are somewhat poorer than those currently obtained.

The results obtained with the fine needle (aspiration cytology) are compared with those obtained with the cutting-edge needle (aspiration biopsy for histologic examination) and other biopsy needles (Tru-Cut). Core biopsies for histologic examination are less frequent in our series than aspirations for cytologic study, because the retrieval of core samples at low risk had to await the development of improved biopsy needles.

The evaluation of fine-needle (Chiba) aspiration biopsies for cytologic diagnosis is oriented toward the malignancy or benignancy of the lesion. Because this type of biopsy was usually done for the purpose of confirming malignancy or investigating a mass uncovered by ultrasound or computed tomography, the final cytologic finding was classified as *true-positive* if the suspected malignancy was confirmed.

A *false-positive* cytologic diagnosis is one that asserts the presence of a malignant tumor where none exists. In reality a false-positive cytologic diagnosis is extremely rare, and we know of only one such case in our experience. There can be false-positive diagnoses with ultrasonography and computed tomography.

A finding is classified as *true-negative* if it demonstrates a benign tissue change where no malignancy exists.

A *false-negative* result is based on inaccurate placement of the biopsy needle (i.e., the needle misses the lesion) or on failure of the cytologist to appreciate the malignant character of the cells (e.g., due to excessive aspiration of blood).

Because *false-positive* results are virtually nonexistent in cytology, we did not generally follow up patients who had a cytologic diagnosis of malignancy. If the cytologic findings were negative, we reviewed the course of the disease on the basis of medical records and statements from attending physicians, provided an inflammatory process (e.g., hepatic abscess, pyonephrosis) could not be inferred from the immediate history. The results were evaluated separately for different organs according to the specificity, sensitivity, and overall success rate of the method.

Table 4. Tissue biopsies

Structures biopsied	n
Liver	527
Kidney/adrenal	247
Pancreas	184
Spleen	12
Retroperitoneal and intraabdominal mass	420
Intestine (including stomach)	48
Gallbladder	5
Ascites	65
Prostate	13
Uterus	5
Bladder	3
Ovary	21
Abdominal wall	19
Solid lung tumor	51
Pleural effusion	93
Solid pleural tumor	30
Mediastinum	13
Pericardium	7
Other (trunk, extremities, soft-tissue lesions near bone)	94
Amniocentesis	17
Thyroid	26
Breast[a]	13
Total	1913

[a] Includes only breasts with nonpalpable parenchymatous or cystic lesions biopsied under sonographic control

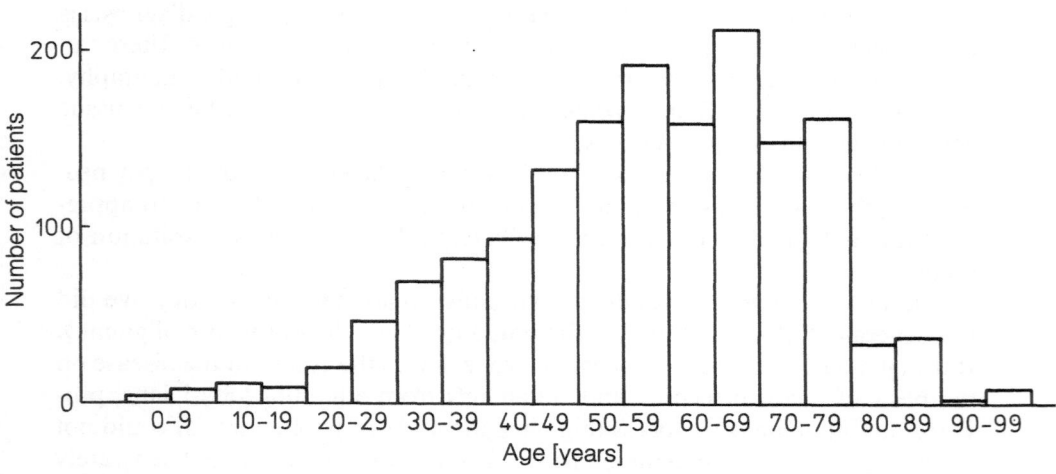

Fig. 27. Age distribution of the 1802 patients biopsied (total of 1913 biopsies: 1056 in men, 857 in women)

1.3 Organs Biopsied

Of the more than 3000 patients biopsied to date, we obtained a cytologic result by fine-needle aspiration biopsy in 1802 (998 men and 804 women) and compared it with the final diagnosis. If multiple biopsies were taken from the same patient on different days, and thus were performed at different sittings, we counted each of them as a separate biopsy. The percentage of these patients is very small. If different sites were biopsied at one sitting (e.g., colon carcinoma with metastasis to the liver), the patient was counted only once, but the biopsies from each region were evaluated separately. This is why the number of biopsies is greater than the number of patients (Table 4).

1.4 Age Distribution

The age distribution is shown in Fig. 27. The youngest patient was a 2½-year-old child, the oldest was 94 years of age.

2 Results of Fine-Needle Aspirations for Specific Organs and Body Regions

2.1 Liver

Biopsy Results for Malignant and Benign Lesions

Years of experience have shown that, in the abdominal region, the liver is the most frequent site of occurrence for sonographically or computed tomographically detected lesions that require further investigation. Formerly, when a focal hepatic lesion was detected by scintigraphy, for example, the only available method of preoperative evaluation was angiography. Aspiration cytology, is more precise and is relatively easy to perform when guided by cross-sectional imaging.

Fine-needle aspiration biopsy was the method most commonly used in our investigations of the liver (Table 5). Of 527 liver biopsies, 294 yielded malignant cells indicative of a primary or metastatic tumor. In 53 patients with hepatic malignancy, a second malignant tumor in the abdomen or thorax was successfully biopsied and identified; these consisted mainly of pancreatic carcinomas, intestinal tumors, and a few bronchial carcinomas.

In eight patients the aspiration of a sonographically localized mass in a region outside the biopsied liver yielded no additional malignant cells, although a malignancy at that location was later confirmed in three of these patients by the subsequent progression of disease. These extrahepatic tumors respectively involved the spleen, kidney, and bladder.

Table 5. Results of fine-needle aspiration biopsies of the liver[a]

Cytologic diagnosis	True-positive	True-negative	False-negative	Total
No. of biopsies	294	214	19	527
(%)	(55.8)	(40.6)	(3.6)	(100)

[a] Evaluation based on "malignant tumor"

Table 6. Focal hepatic lesions not identifiable with ultrasound that proved to be benign

Lesions	n
Hepatic abscesses	44
Hepatic hemangiomas	28
Hepatic cysts	26
Benign tumors (adenomas)	
Focal hyperplasias	
Regnerative nodules	
Focal steatoses, etc.	116
Total	214

Nineteen patients had malignant liver tumors that were not initially diagnosed. Most of these were richly vascularized primary tumors in which considerable blood had been aspirated along with the cancer cells, or a definitive cytologic diagnosis could not be made because of the similarity of normal hepatocytes to tumor cells.

Because of this, we now biopsy the liver with a thin cutting-edge needle whenever there is clinical suspicion of a hepatic tumor, even when the cytologic findings are negative. While this technique will not diagnose all malignant tumors in all patients, it provides a higher accuracy than aspiration cytology.

In 214 patients the liver biopsy findings indicated a benign space-occupying lesion (Table 6). In 13 patients the second, extrahepatic biopsy indicated a malignancy even though the liver biopsy yielded only benign cells.

In a total of 39 patients, the result of the cytologic examination did not correlate with ultrasound findings, and further evaluation was not possible because the patients were lost to follow-up. We excluded this group when calculating the accuracy of the method.

The following accuracy rates, with allowance for possible errors in the cytology laboratory, were calculated for the hepatic fine-needle aspiration biopsies in our series (see Table 5):

Specificity	100%,
Sensitivity	91%,
Overall success rate	96.4%.

In spite of the generally good results of fine-needle aspiration biopsy of the liver, the 91% sensitivity of the method is markedly below the values for retroperitoneal tumors or pancreatic carcinoma, although other authors report similar figures for it [15, 72, 101, 152]. This may have some connection with patient selection, since we attempted to biopsy even small and very small lesions that were visible sonographically. Also, there are methodological limitations of the procedure and practical difficulties of specimen collection with an aspiration needle (see Sects. A 2.2 and A 3.4).

An accurate cytologic diagnosis cannot be made if the quality of the aspirate is poor. This may occur in association with the problems listed below and can limit the value of fine-needle aspiration biopsies of other organs as well:

Special Problems of Fine-Needle Aspiration Biopsy

1. Richly vascularized tumor: Aspiration of blood, which masks the tumor cells
2. Very small tumor (< 1 cm): For physical reasons, difficult to reach with a fine needle
3. Heavily fibrotic tumor: Inadequate cellular material
4. Uncooperative patient: Small lesions cannot be aspirated unless respiration is suspended

With strongly vascularized tumors and expansive, fibrotic processes, the diagnostic yield can be improved by modifying the tactics of the biopsy. Thus the aspiration of blood can be reduced by applying less suction to the needle. Also, puncturing the lesion with a short, jabbing movement of the needle (harpoon technique) can provide basically site-specific cell material. This technique has proved effective with hemangiomas as well as with primary liver tumors such as hepatocytic adenoma. The use of a thin cutting-edge needle has proved advantageous, for it is somewhat more rigid than the fine aspiration needle and therefore easier to guide in tissue, yet it is flexible enough to prevent laceration of the liver capsule. Even the typical endothelial cells of hemangioma are easily aspirated with the smallest-caliber cutting-edge needle. The rare hamartoma of the liver is biopsied in the same way; usually benign histiocytes are obtained.

Poor cooperation by the patient cannot be remedied by a simple modification of technique. However, local anesthesia prior to fine-needle aspiration biopsy, while not routine, may make the procedure easier to tolerate as it accustoms the patient to the pain of the needle and deadens the peritoneum.

Limiting ultrasound-guided biopsy to certain regions of the liver, most notably the subdiaphragmatic portion of the right lobe, is recommended by some authors [140] but does not appear justified in practice. With correct sonographic technique, the entire liver can be well visualized even with a linear-array transducer. Also, there is a trend toward the use of combination systems that include a sector scanner.

It is important to note that even a fine-needle aspiration of the liver may stimulate the vagus nerve, with cardiac arrest as the most serious potential consequence. In our experience this phenomenon is very rare and, we believe, is most apt to occur when the needle pierces structures in the region of the hilus and hepatic duct.

2.2 Retroperitoneal and Intraperitoneal Masses

Despite advances in technique, the retroperitoneum was long considered a difficult region for ultrasound evaluation, and even today computed tomography is justifiably considered the principal modality for evaluations of retroperitoneal structures. With improvements in real-time sonographic technique, structures such as the pancreas, aorta, and inferior vena cava could be imaged with increasing accuracy and detail, and soon the ultrasound-guided fine-needle aspiration of tumors in this region became practical.

At the very start of the ultrasound era, the kidneys could be accurately evaluated. They are located more superficially, and the relatively sonolucent liver and spleen provide good acoustic windows for the imaging of renal tissue.

The sonographic identification of the adrenals continues to be a problem. Normal-sized adrenals can be consistently demonstrated only in computed tomography scans, although visualization of the adrenals with ultrasound has been reported. Tumors 2 cm or more in diameter can usually be visualized when a specific search is made. Adrenal hyperplasia, on the other hand, can be diagnosed only by angiography or computed tomography.

A separate section is devoted to the pancreas (see below), because that organ occupies a unique place in terms of diagnosis and treatment. Also, its relatively anterior position and the presence of echogenic landmarks such as the splenic vein and the confluence of the splenic vein and superior mesenteric vein make it easily accessible to sonography.

The main contingent for ultrasound-guided biopsies of retroperitoneal structures is enlarged lymph nodes as a manifestation of metastatic or lymphomatous disease.

Besides the focal liver changes previously discussed, intraperitoneal masses include focal lesions of the spleen, which are somewhat uncommon. We have mainly biopsied enlarged intraperitoneal lymph nodes at the hepatic portal, at the origin of the visceral branches of the great vessels, and elsewhere. Most were manifestations of a malignant lymphoma, and a few were metastatic.

Data on the success rates of biopsies of intra- and retroperitoneal masses are very encouraging. It should be noted, however, that ultrasound-guided fine-needle aspiration biopsies were performed in a patient group only after computed tomograms had first been obtained. In particular, tumors associated with Hodgkin's disease tend to be small and can be difficult to localize with ultrasound alone.

A total of 420 intraperitoneal or retroperitoneal masses located outside the large parenchymatous organs were biopsied. This group did not include tumors

Table 7. Results of fine-needle aspiration biopsies of retro- and intraperitoneal masses

Cytologic diagnosis	True-positive	True-negative	False-negative	Total
No. of patients	191	169	38	398
(%)	(48)	(42.5)	(9.5)	(100)

of the lesser pelvis or bowel. The results of 398 biopsies could be accurately evaluated (Table 7).

Malignant cells were recovered from 191 patients, or slightly less than half of all patients in the group. Definitive evidence of malignancy was obtained in 229 patients. Eighteen patients had neoplasms coexisting with their intra- or retroperitoneal tumors, most involving the liver.

The cytologic result, and thus presumably the biopsy, was *false-negative* in 38 patients. Malignant disease was later confirmed in these patients although the aspiration did not yield tumor cells.

Benign changes were present in 169 patients, as confirmed by clinical follow-up, surgery, or other examinations.

While most of the malignant tumors were lymphomas (Hodgkin's or non-Hodgkin's lymphoma), metastases (mainly testicular tumors), and primary tumors, the most frequent benign masses were inflammatory changes of lymph nodes, abscesses, and hematomas.

Looking at the success rates, we find that they are somewhat lower on average than those of the liver biopsies: Sensitivity is 83.4%, specificity is 100%, and the overall success rate is 90.5%, assuming that only the detection of malignant tumors constitutes a true-positive result. This is not entirely satisfactory, however, because there were many cases in which the clinical presentation and history were consistent with a hematoma or abscess, but not with a malignant tumor.

2.3 Pancreas

Biopsy Results for Malignant and Benign Lesions

The pancreas was biopsied in more than 200 patients. In 184 cases the cytologic result was compared with the clinical course or with the final diagnosis at surgery or autopsy. In ten cases a definitive diagnosis could not be made.

The smallest tumor biopsied was 1.6 cm in diameter. It was detected relatively early because of its association with obstructive jaundice. In our opinion it is very unusual for a solid pancreatic lesion less than 2 cm in diameter to be identified. It remains to be seen whether endocavitary (e.g., endogastric) ultrasound techniques will contribute to the routine detection of smaller pancreatic tumors.

Of 174 patients with malignant pancreatic tumors, cytologic findings were positive in 106. This corresponds to 60.9% of all subsequently confirmed malig-

Table 8. Diagnosis of malignant pancreatic tumors

Cytologic diagnosis	True-positive	True-negative	False-negative	Total
Number of biopsies	106	57	11	174
(%)	(60.9)	(32.8)	(6.3)	(100)

nancies (Table 8). In one patient with a fist-sized tumor of the tail of the pancreas, a diagnosis of hypernephroma was initially presumed from the sonographic picture.

In five patients the aspirate from coexisting hepatic tumors that appeared to be metastatic was found to contain malignant cells, but tumor cells were not recovered from the pancreas itself. Nevertheless, in 94.6% of the patients a pancreatic neoplasm was identified by sonography or cytology as the probable origin of the tumor. In 19 patients malignant cells were recovered both from the pancreatic region and from the liver in separate aspirations.

There were no false-positive diagnoses, and so the specificity in this group was 100%. True-negative diagnoses were made in 57 patients. Chronic pancreatitis was known to be present in the majority. Biopsy was done for the purpose of differentiating a circumscribed, inflammatory organ enlargement from a tumor.

In 11 patients aspiration biopsy yielded no malignant cells despite later confirmation of a pancreatic carcinoma. This corresponds to a false-negative rate of 6.3%.

Overall, we obtained the following accuracy rates in fine-needle aspirations of the pancreas:

Specificity 100%,
Sensitivity 90.6% pancreatic tumors alone
(94.9% pancreatic tumors or hepatic metastases with sonographic evidence of a pancreatic lesion),
Overall success rate 93.7%.

Evaluation of Pancreatic Fine-Needle Aspiration

Although computed tomography and sonography have not led to an early diagnosis of pancreatic carcinoma and thus have done little to improve survival rates in these patients, the cross-sectional imaging methods are very helpful in the evaluation of patients with unexplained abdominal pain and occasionally permit an early, definitive diagnosis to be made.

Not every space-occupying lesion of the pancreas is a carcinoma. Pancreatitis, especially when chronic, is at times accompanied by tumor-like changes that mimic a neoplasm but in reality represent pseudocysts with detritus or possibly a solid tissue swelling.

Because malignant tumors occasionally incite an inflammatory reaction, a positive cytologic diagnosis of pancreatic carcinoma will be missed in a small percentage of patients. The false-negative rate is substantially higher when the organ is surgically exposed for biopsy, for it is usually difficult to identify the center of the tumor. This is a strong argument against the claim that fine-needle aspiration biopsy is unnecessary in suspected pancreatic cancer owing to the availability of intraoperative biopsy. It is in the patient's best interests to decide before surgery whether it is better to perform a definitive resection with curative intent or select a palliative procedure such as internal drainage with bypass of the tumor stenosis.

Not all space-occupying lesions at the level of the pancreas arise from that organ. Thus one of our patients with macromorphological evidence of pancreatic carcinoma was found to have metastatic tumors that arose from an ovarian carcinoma and were simply displacing the pancreas. In two other patients we found enlarged lymph nodes that had undergone reactive changes.

The enlarged caudate lobe in hepatic cirrhosis can also mimic a pancreatic tumor, especially if coexisting ascites makes it difficult to visualize the retroperitoneal area.

As mentioned earlier, one patient was diagnosed by ultrasound as having a hypernephroma, an approximately fist-sized tumor that appeared to arise from the cranial pole of the left kidney. Fine-needle aspiration proved that the lesion was not a hypernephroma, as the procedure yielded malignant cells indicative of a tumor metastatic to the pancreas or a primary pancreatic carcinoma. The presence of such a malignant tumor was confirmed at operation, at which time it was found that the tumor had indeed infiltrated the left renal capsule.

Contamination of the aspirate by blood can make cytologic evaluation difficult. If the pancreatic tumor is found to coexist with lesions suggestive of hepatic metastases, it is recommended that the suspected metastases also be biopsied, as this will increase the reliability of the diagnosis and aid in making a prognosis. It will also help to determine what form of therapy is indicated, e.g., surgical resection, a bypass operation, or percutaneous drainage.

The fine-needle aspiration biopsy of pancreatic tumors offers various advantages to the patient and physician. It has significantly shortened the time needed to diagnose this disease, as Fig. 28 demonstrates. In some cases a diagnosis can be established very quickly, and the biopsy may even be done as an outpatient procedure. This saves a great deal of time and obviates the need for more invasive diagnostic studies.

According to our evaluation, coexisting hepatic metastases were detected by aspiration biopsy in 19 patients with malignant cells of the pancreatic region. This represents 16.3% of the 117 patients in whom a final diagnosis of pancreatic carcinoma was confirmed. If we add to this the five patients in whom malignant cells were aspirated from hepatic metastases but not from the suspicious pancreatic lesion noted on sonograms, the percentage of tumors that had metastasized by the time of their discovery rises to 20.5%. Even when sonographic

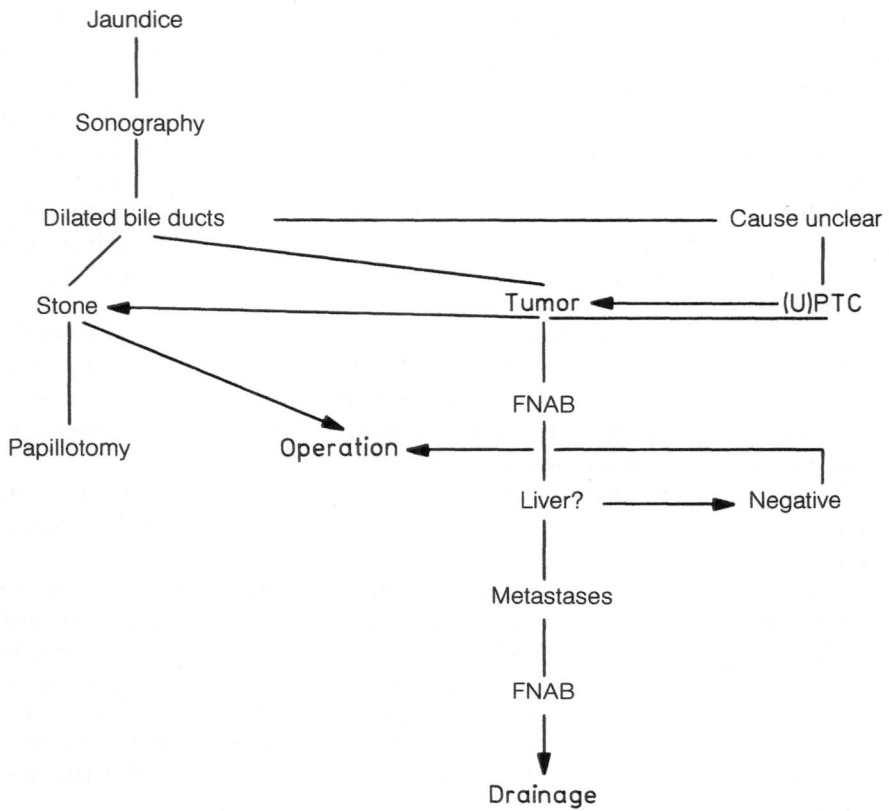

Fig. 28. Flowchart for the evaluation of jaundice. *FNAB,* fine-needle aspiration biopsy; *(U)PTC* ultrasound-guided percutaneous transhepatic cholangiography

criteria are applied, cancer of the pancreas is often so far advanced at the time of its detection that curative therapy is no longer possible.

A number of authors have published data on the diagnostic accuracy of pancreatic fine-needle aspiration biopsies (Table 9). Various methods of tumor localization were employed. The exact sensitivity and specificity rates were recalculated so that they could be more easily compared with our data [17]. As the table indicates, the highest accuracy rates were achieved at our institute. This result is not surprising, for our strict adherence to correct biopsy technique (aspiration of cells from the tumor periphery rather than from the degenerate center, repeat aspiration if the initial sample contained too much blood, use of cutting-edge needles, immediate fixation in Delauney solution by trained personnel, etc.) ensured a maximum yield of diagnostic material.

We observed no significant complications following pancreatic biopsy. After the inadequate aspiration of fluid from a pancreatic pseudocyst, one patient complained of transient epigastric pain that lasted about an hour. Presumably

Table 9. Diagnostic accuracy of pancreatic biopsy

Author:	Schwerk [151]	Braun [15]	Mitty [112]	Hodenak [70]	Holm [72]	Klahn [85]	Our results
No. of biopsies	50	63	53	55	205	79	164
Diagnostic accuracy (%)	(90)	(96,8)	(88,7)	(81,3)	(92,7)	(94,9)	(92,8)
Sensitivity (%)	(84,6)	(92,6)	(86)	(77,3)	(79)	(85,7)	(89)
Specificity (%)	(100)	(100)	(100)	(100)	(100)	(100)	(100)

this was caused by leakage of cystic fluid through the needle tract into the abdomen. Late complications did not occur.

Necrotizing pancreatitis precipitated by biopsy is described in the literature. But in cases of pancreatitis or a pancreatic tumor, it is safe to assume that the disease has damaged the organ far more than the fine-needle aspiration. Endoscopic retrograde pancreatography is considered more dangerous in terms of the risk of necrotizing pancreatitis.

2.4 Gastrointestinal Tumors

Special Case of the Sonography of an Intestinal Tumor

By its nature, sonography is not an acceptable screening method for detecting tumors of the gastrointestinal tract. Occasionally, however, a tumor involving the body of the stomach, the wall of the antrum, or the colon may be so extensive that it presents as a circumscribed wall thickening or abnormal mass on sonograms and can therefore be biopsied under direct vision.

Percutaneous biopsies of the intestinal tract at our center account for only a small percentage of the whole. But because the procedure is very simple and economical, and because it sometimes eliminates the need for more costly diagnostic studies, it is worth mentioning in relation to the investigation of certain gastrointestinal masses.

The distal body of the stomach and the antrum normally present as a thin, ring-like structure located below or behind the visceral surface of the liver and anterior to the superior mesenteric artery and vein and the pancreas. The normal colon is only occasionally delineated as a ring-like structure. For examination of the colon, the ultrasound transducer is moved continuously over the abdomen, following the course of the large intestine, recognized by the presence of hyperechoic zones (gas content!). Although the bowel usually cannot be imaged over its entire extent, this study nevertheless allows pathologic findings to be localized grossly to a particular colonic segment.

In the recumbent patient the cecum and flexures are easily delineated by ultrasound owing to their gaseous contents. The examination is performed without special preparatory measures. The patient does not need to fast, although the bladder should be filled if possible to aid evaluation of disease arising from the rectosigmoid.

Because the likelihood of detecting a primary gastrointestinal tumor with the cross-sectional imaging methods is not very high – only rectal carcinoma is relatively easy to diagnose with computed tomography – a true screening examination of the middle and lower abdomen for gastrointestinal disease was rarely performed. This might be indicated only if there were a high index of suspicion for such disease or if hepatic metastases were detected whose cytologic picture was consistent with colorectal carcinoma.

Technique of Tumor Wall Biopsy

Gastric and intestinal tumors are characterized in sonograms by an eccentric thickening of the wall, which also appears rigid. A strong, broad, central echo signifies an intraluminal collection of gas, which often appears immobile, and this feature is consistent with classic tumor findings.

The sight line of the biopsy transducer is directed toward the center of the tumor. With moderate wall thickening, the needle is inserted somewhat tangentially and eccentrically with respect to the side wall. This will increase the length of tumor-involved bowel wall traversed by the biopsy needle and improve the chance of aspirating tumor cells.

The biopsy is performed with a fine cytology needle, because cutting-edge needles carry a greater risk of hemorrhage or even perforation of the already damaged bowel wall.

Results

A total of 32 intestinal tumors and three perityphlitic abscesses were investigated by biopsy. Malignant cells indicative of adenocarcinoma were identified in 26 patients. Remarkably, cytologic findings were negative in six patients with intestinal cancer. This may be due to an inflammatory reaction of adjacent mucosal areas or to the very firm consistency of connective-tissue-rich tumors, from which adequate cellular material cannot be collected with the fine Chiba needle.

By its nature, sonography can identify an infiltrative lesion of the gastric or bowel wall as being malignant only if there is coexisting evidence of malignancy such as hepatic metastases or obvious expansion of the tumor into the mesentery. If these findings are not present, a malignant wall tumor cannot be confidently distinguished from an inflammatory or cicatricial wall lesion.

The relatively high false-negative rate in our series (including cytologist errors) is explained in part by the difficulty of impaling tubular, often easily displaced intestinal structures with the relatively blunt aspiration needle. The absence of complications is consistent with the experience of other investigators [40, 147].

56

It should be reemphasized that sonography is not an acceptable screening technique for intestinal tumors; it is rewarding only when neoplastic disease is advanced. Radiologic contrast studies of the digestive tract remain the mainstay of noninvasive diagnosis. They are equivalent to invasive endoscopy in the localization of involved gastrointestinal segments and are even superior to endoscopy in general evaluations of the gastrointestinal tract (small intestine!), but they do not provide material for histologic study.

Despite the limitations of sonography, we believe that its many advantages justify its use, possibly combined with ultrasound-guided aspiration biopsy, as a first-line measure for the early evaluation of undiagnosed abdominal disease or palpable abdominal masses. Simply and noninvasively, ultrasound yields valuable information on the large parenchymatous organs of the upper abdomen, as illustrated by its ability to detect colon carcinoma metastatic to the liver. It must be considered, moreover, that an ultrasound examination can be made difficult or impossible by the previous administration of barium.

2.5 Extraabdominal Organs

Intrathoracic Masses

While sonographic techniques have long been used routinely for evaluations of pregnancy and the abdomen in general, some years passed before an attempt was made to utilize ultrasound for examinations of the thoracic region. Because of the large impedance difference that exists between the chest wall and aerated lung, most of the energy of the ultrasound beam is reflected at the pleural interface. As a result, intrathoracic organs other than the heart are not normally accessible to ultrasound evaluation.

Nevertheless, ultrasonography is able to provide much useful information on diseases affecting the lung and pleura [79]. Thus, for example, a pleural effusion is readily distinguished from a pleural thickening or solid tumor. Lung tumors that extend to the periphery can also be identified if they are large enough and are abutted intercostally to the chest wall. However, ultrasound is still less effective than computed tomography when it comes to classifying the tumor as malignant or benign.

If an intrathoracic expansive process is sufficiently large and extends into the mediastinum, it can be traced to that point sonographically. It is expected that endoesophageal sonography will permit an even more accurate identification of such tumors in the future.

In patients who have undergone pneumonectomy, sonography can be used in selected cases to differentiate between a fibrothorax and a centrally located recurrent tumor.

Just as in the abdomen, ultrasound-guided fine-needle aspiration biopsy is an important adjunct in the evaluation of intrathoracic disease, whether for aspirating (or draining) an encapsulated effusion, collecting cells from a solid tumor, or identifying a pleural mesothelioma where chest-wall fibrosis second-ary to tuberculosis was presumed.

Special Biopsy Problems. Before the advent of cross-sectional imaging methods, lung biopsies were performed exclusively with the use of fluoroscopic control [51, 145, 171].

For suspected peripheral tumors that have infiltrated the chest wall, computed tomography may also be used to direct the biopsy. Centrally located masses, however, should not be biopsied by this method, which is time-consuming and carries an increased risk of pneumothorax.

If possible, fine-needle aspiration biopsy should be performed in the supine patient after first positioning the sight line of the transducer on the area of interest. Although the procedural details of the intrathoracic biopsy are very similar to those of abdominal biopsies, some distinctions should be noted:

1. Pneumothorax is always a potential danger, because it is sometimes difficult to determine beforehand whether the lesion is pleural-based or intrapulmonary.
2. Because of respiratory excursions, lesions of the diaphragm are particularly difficult to biopsy.
3. Respiration must be suspended when the biopsy is taken.
4. During respiratory excursions, the needle tip echo will become lost behind a rib unless the transducer is well positioned in an intercostal space.
5. The curvature of the chest reduces the area of transducer contact and thus the size of the image field.

As in traditional lung biopsies under fluoroscopic control, we follow the ultrasound- or computed-tomography-guided biopsy with a chest radiograph to exclude incipient pneumothorax. Depending on the result, the patient may be kept under clinical observation for another 4 h so that any progression of the pneumothorax will be recognized.

Needles for Lung Biopsy. The standard Chiba fine needle is the instrument of choice for biopsies of intrathoracic masses that are visible sonographically. With its small diameter and sharp tip, this disposable needle causes minimal trauma to tissues and lessens the danger of pneumothorax. With a pleural-based lesion that is adherent to the chest wall, a larger-caliber needle may safely be used (see p. 40). The Rotex needle is also a useful instrument but requires more time to take the specimen. This "more invasive" needle is associated with a higher incidence of pneumothorax, as described in the literature [75], yet it furnishes only enough material for cytologic evaluation. It is very difficult to make a smear with this needle, because cellular material tends to become trapped in the grooves of the helical stylet.

We prefer to use a cutting-edge needle for biopsies of fixed pleural tumors or intrapulmonary masses that are abutted to the chest wall. Of course, this in-

Table 10. Results of intrathoracic biopsy with fine needle for cytology/bacteriology and with cutting-edge needle for histology (n = 194)

	Benign	Malignant	Unclear	Inflammatory	Total
Parenchymal lung tumor	8	29	–	14	51
Pleural effusion	41	29	1	22	93[a]
Solid pleural tumor	12	17	1	–	30
Mediastinal tumor[b]	4 (+2 false-negative)	7	–	–	13
Pericardial lesion	7 (6 pericardial effusions, 1 lipoma)	–	–	–	7
	72	82	2	36	194

[a] Without drainage
[b] Including lymph nodes and posterior mediastinum (see Fig. 34)

strument is somewhat more invasive than a fine aspiration needle, and the advantage of obtaining a histologic specimen must be weighed against the increased risk of pneumothorax.

Results. Of 366 patients who underwent percutaneous aspiration or core biopsies of the thoracic region, we were able to compare the cellular or tissue material with subsequent findings at follow-up, surgery, or autopsy in 194.

As Table 10 indicates, the results in two of these patients could not be classified. Of the remaining 192 patients, a malignant intrathoracic tumor or malignant metastasis was demonstrated in 82 (42.7%). An inflammatory process was diagnosed in 36 patients (18.8%). The majority of the patients who were not followed up and were not included in the table had inflammatory and noninflammatory pleural effusions, some probably secondary to pulmonary embolism. Seventeen of the patients in whom cytologic findings were negative were subsequently identified as having a malignant tumor.

Biopsies of mediastinal tumors present a special challenge, due largely to the risk of inadvertent vascular puncture when the procedure is done under fluoroscopic or computed tomographic control. Thus, ultrasound guidance is preferred for mediastinal biopsies if the lesion can be clearly delineated, though often this is not possible because of intervening aerated lung. Below we present two examples illustrating the use of intrathoracic biopsy under sonographic guidance. The first patient was a 27-year-old woman with peripheral neoplasia close to the chest wall; the second was a 39-year-old man with a small mass in the posteroinferior mediastinum. The possibility of using computed tomography to direct fine-needle aspiration biopsies will not be discussed here.

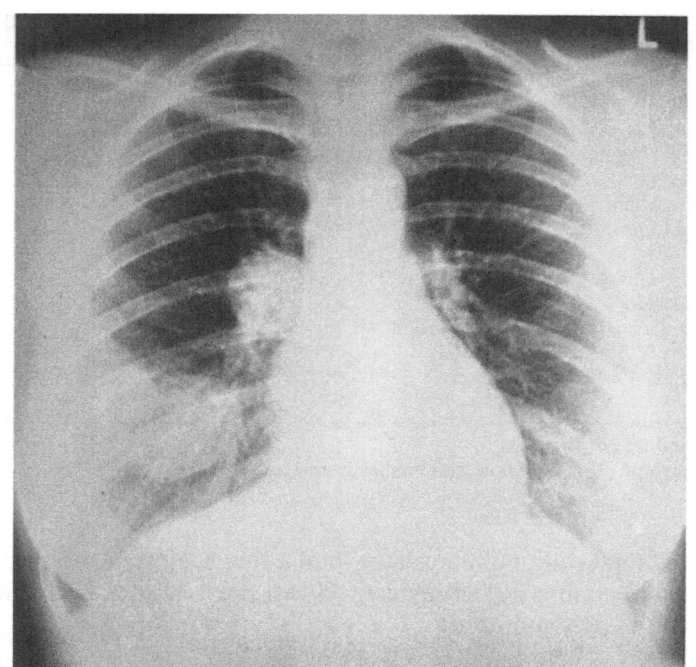

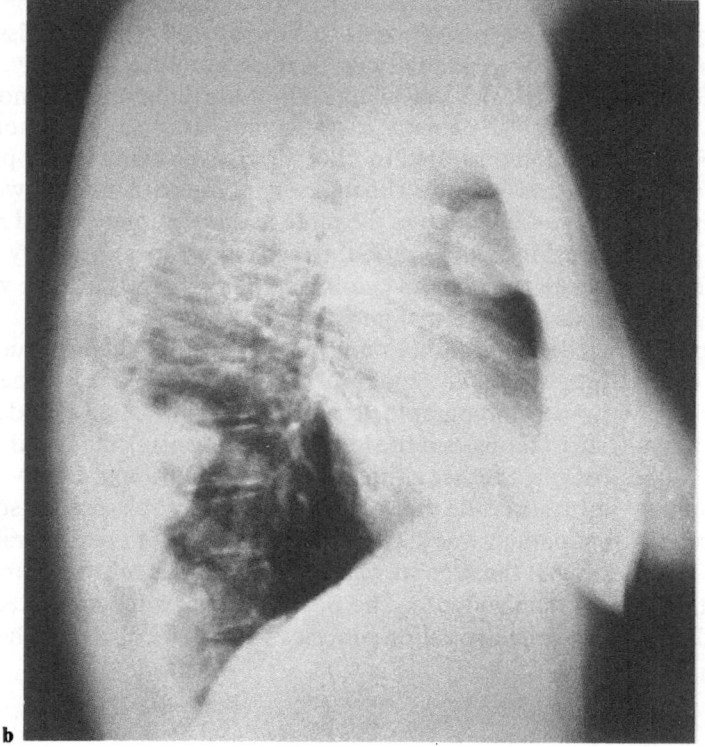

60

Case Reports

Example 1 of intrathoracic biopsy under sonographic control:

A nurse born in 1957 complained of pain in the right half of the thorax that was most pronounced posteriorly. Initial laboratory tests showed only an elevation of the erythrocyte sedimentation rate. Chest films demonstrated two fairly large, rounded masses in the right half of the thorax; the lateral projection showed that one was located anteriorly and one far posteriorly. The radiographic presentation was consistent with tumor masses, possibly pleural metastases (Fig. 29 a,b). Ultrasound scans of the abdomen were unrewarding. Subsequent computed tomographic scans reinforced the impression of two pleural-based masses in the right half of the thorax (Fig. 30).

Next we performed an ultrasound-guided biopsy with a small-caliber (0.95-mm) cutting-edge needle (Fig. 31). The procedure was well tolerated, and the biopsy specimen was referred for histologic evaluation. A pathologic diagnosis of sarcoma was returned (Fig. 32), and this was confirmed at operation. The lesion abutting on the anterior chest wall was judged to be metastatic; no additional tumor involvement was noted.

The preparation in Fig. 32 shows that the cutting-edge needle can retrieve material that is useful for histologic evaluation. The figure shows the full diameter of the tissue core but only a portion of its length, which can easily reach 3 cm when proper technique is used.

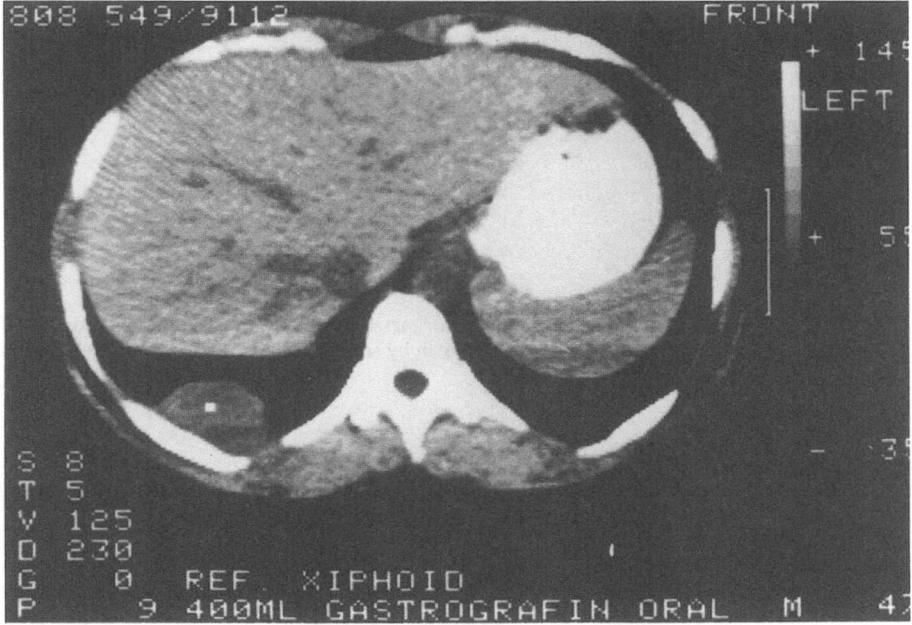

Fig. 30. Computed tomographic scan demonstrates a posterocaudal mass near the pleura in the right half of the thorax

Fig. 29 a,b. Chest radiograph. **a** Anteroposterior film shows two smooth-bordered masses in the right half of the chest. **b** Lateral film demonstrates the two masses in proximity to the chest wall

61

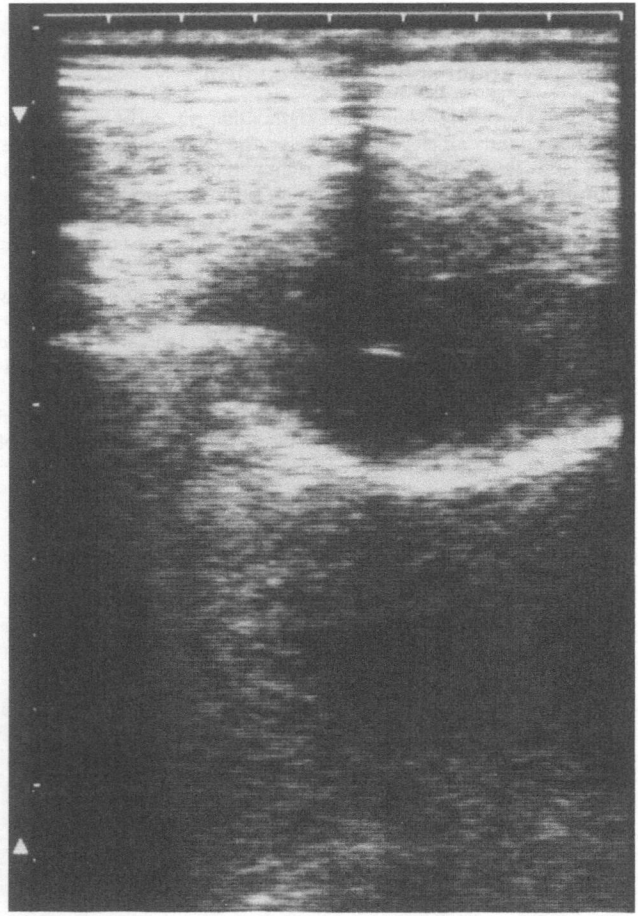

Fig. 31. Ultrasound-guided biopsy of the posterior mass in Fig. 30 with a thin cutting-edge needle. The intrapulmonary location of the tumor is shown by sonographic monitoring (marked displacement with respiration)

Example 2: Ultrasound-guided biopsy of the posterior mediastinum through an anterior approach:

Colectomy for familial polyposis became necessary in a 39-year-old man. Four years previously, several lymph nodes in the surgical specimen had shown carcinomatous degeneration, but no metastases had been found.

The patient now consulted a rheumatologist with pain in the left sacrum, and diagnostic studies included computed tomographic scans. Because a slight elevation of previously normal CEA values (carcinoembryonic antigen) had recently been noted, computed tomography scans of the upper abdomen were also obtained. These revealed a small, nodular mass in the posteroinferior mediastinum just above the crura of the diaphragm (Fig. 33). A previous ultrasound examination had failed to delineate this lesion. After it was localized by computed tomography, it could also be documented with a sector ultrasound scan (Fig. 34).

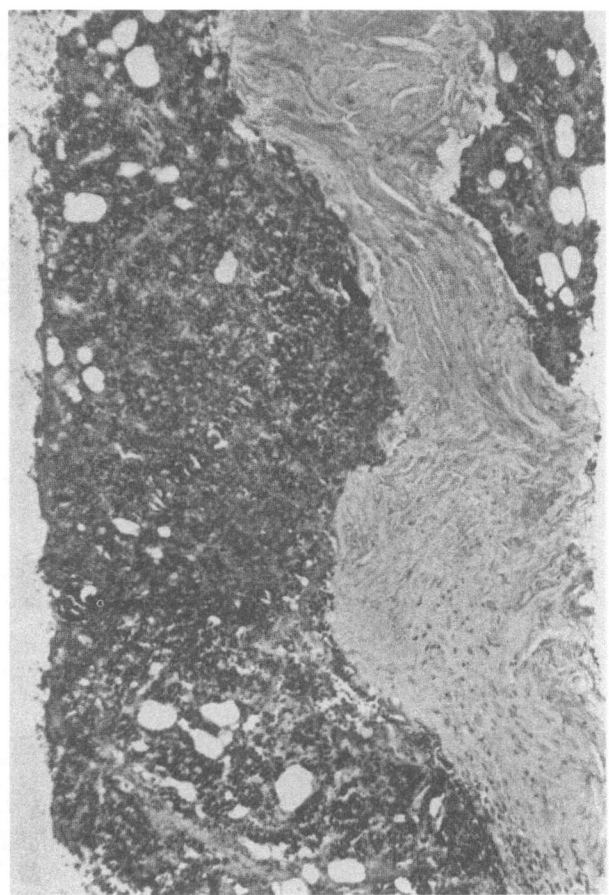

Fig. 32. Macroscopic preparation of the tissue core obtained with the cutting-edge needle: extraosseous osteosarcoma!

The corresponding "target scan" with the linear-array transducer demonstrated the mass as a small, flattened oval situated anterior to the spine (Fig. 35). It projected behind the inferior vena cava. In that position the mass could be biopsied. Figure 36 shows the Chiba-type needle deviating in a slightly cranial direction; the echogenic needle tip is visible within the tumor at the bottom of the picture. Cytologic investigation revealed cells from a colon carcinoma metastatic to the mediastinum.

Cervical Region

The cervical region is a frequent site of findings which warrant fine-needle aspiration biopsy. Two broad categories of patients may be distinguished: those with a palpable thyroid nodule, and those with enlarged lymph nodes.

Most thyroid nodules are readily palpated, making it easy to aspirate material and prepare a smear [33]. There are exceptions, however. The accurate localization of a nodule can be difficult if it is very soft or deeply situated, or espe-

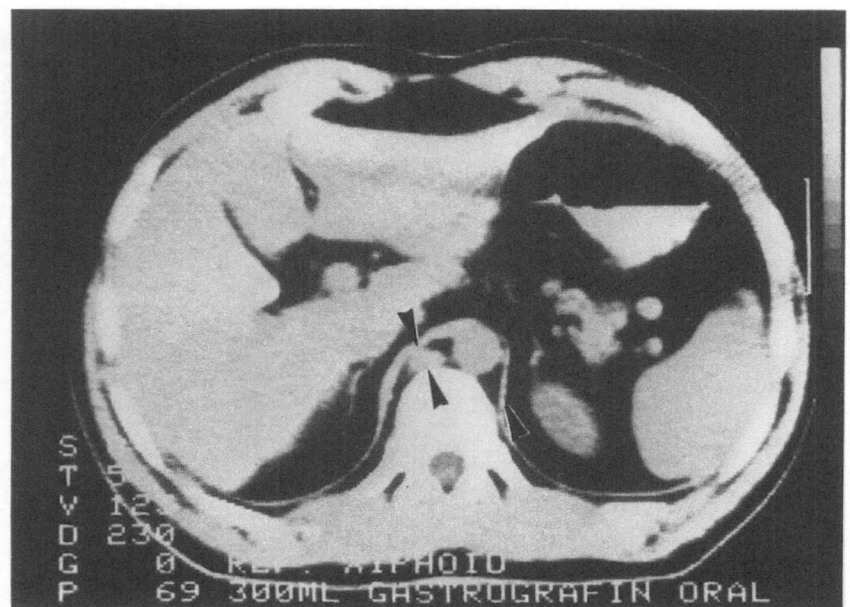

Fig. 33. Computed tomographic scan through the upper abdomen demonstrates a small, nodular mass behind the right crus of the diaphragm and immediately anterior to the spine *(arrows)*. The appearance of the lesion is consistent with a solitary metastasis of the posteroinferior mediastinum

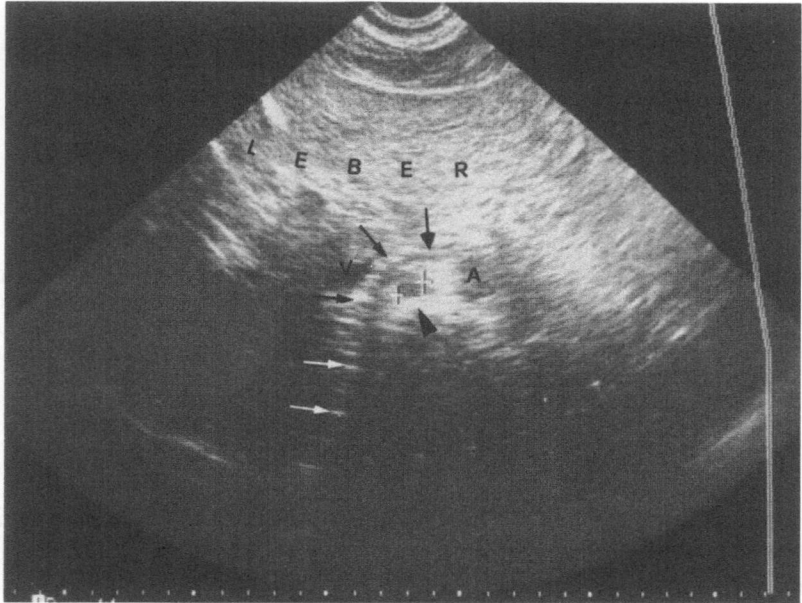

Fig. 34. Transverse sector scan of the same plane (and same patient) as in Fig. 33. The juxtaaortic tumor is marked with a *large arrow*, and its size is indicated by *crosses* (11 mm). *A*, aorta; *V*, inferior vena cava; *small arrow*, right crus of diaphragm

64

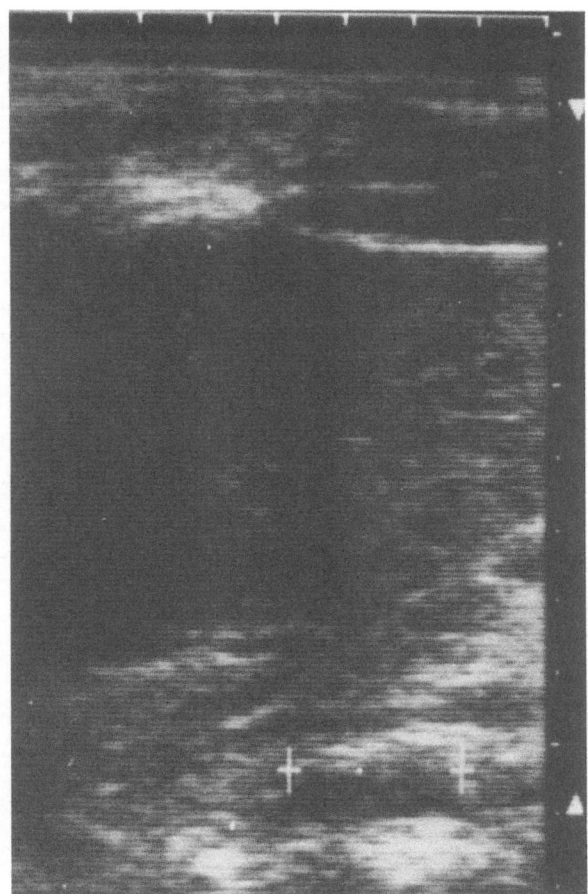

Fig. 35. Longitudinal scan through the prevertebral tumor. The tumor measures about 1 cm in the sagittal direction and about 2 cm in the longitudinal direction *(marks)*

cially if the gland is retrosternal. In these few cases it is safer to perform the aspiration under ultrasound guidance.

At our center, a clearly palpable thyroid nodule is biopsied by a skilled cytologist in accordance with clinical findings. We use ultrasound guidance only in exceptional cases, as when isotope scans reveal a cold nodule that is nonpalpable. In practical terms, the diagnostic value of routine thyroid aspiration biopsy is limited by the difficulty of excluding more highly differentiated tumors by aspiration cytology. Increasingly, we are turning to the use of thin cutting-edge needles (diameter 0.95 mm) for biopsies of the thyroid.

While most palpable masses of the cervical region are biopsied without difficulty, there are exceptions. Thus, there have been instances where patients referred to us from the ear, nose, and throat department had undergone repeated aspirations of palpable masses without recovery of useful cell material. One such patient had a firm mass in the right cervical area following radiation thera-

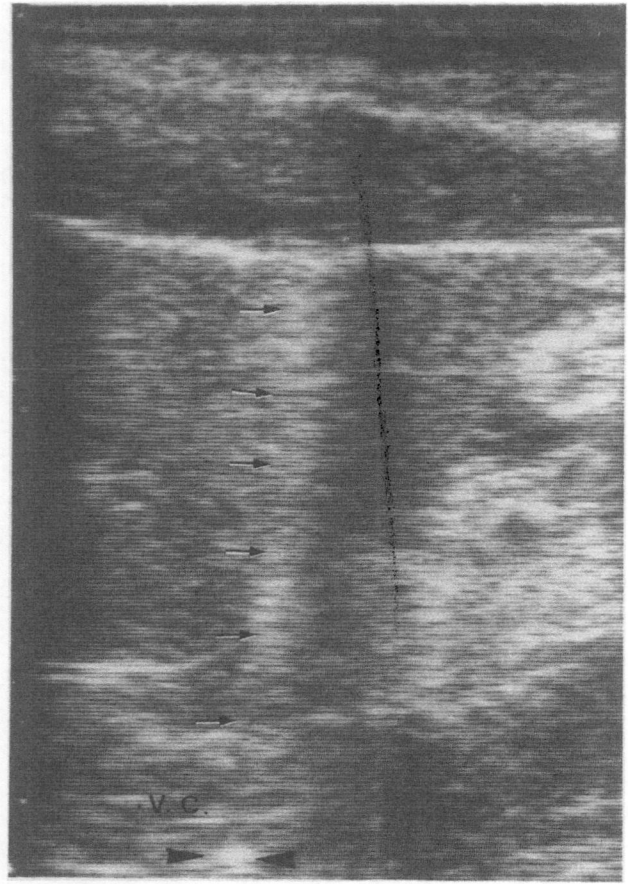

Fig. 36. Moment of ultrasound-guided fine-needle aspiration (image is faint because photo was taken from videotape). There is a slight craniad *(right-to-left)* deviation of the needle in the liver. The vena cava *(V. C.)* is compressed and has been pierced by the aspiration needle. The needle tip appears as a bright echo *(large arrows)*; the *small arrows* mark the shaft

py (Fig. 37 a,b). The centrally degenerate tumor (a metastasis from lung carcinoma) was immediately demonstrated with ultrasound in the fibrotic cervical soft tissues and was directly biopsied.

Blind aspiration biopsy is sometimes unsuccessful in cellulitic lesions as well, because the peripheral abscess is often very thin and narrow and difficult to localize clinically. With ultrasound, the depth of the pus collection can usually be determined with great accuracy.

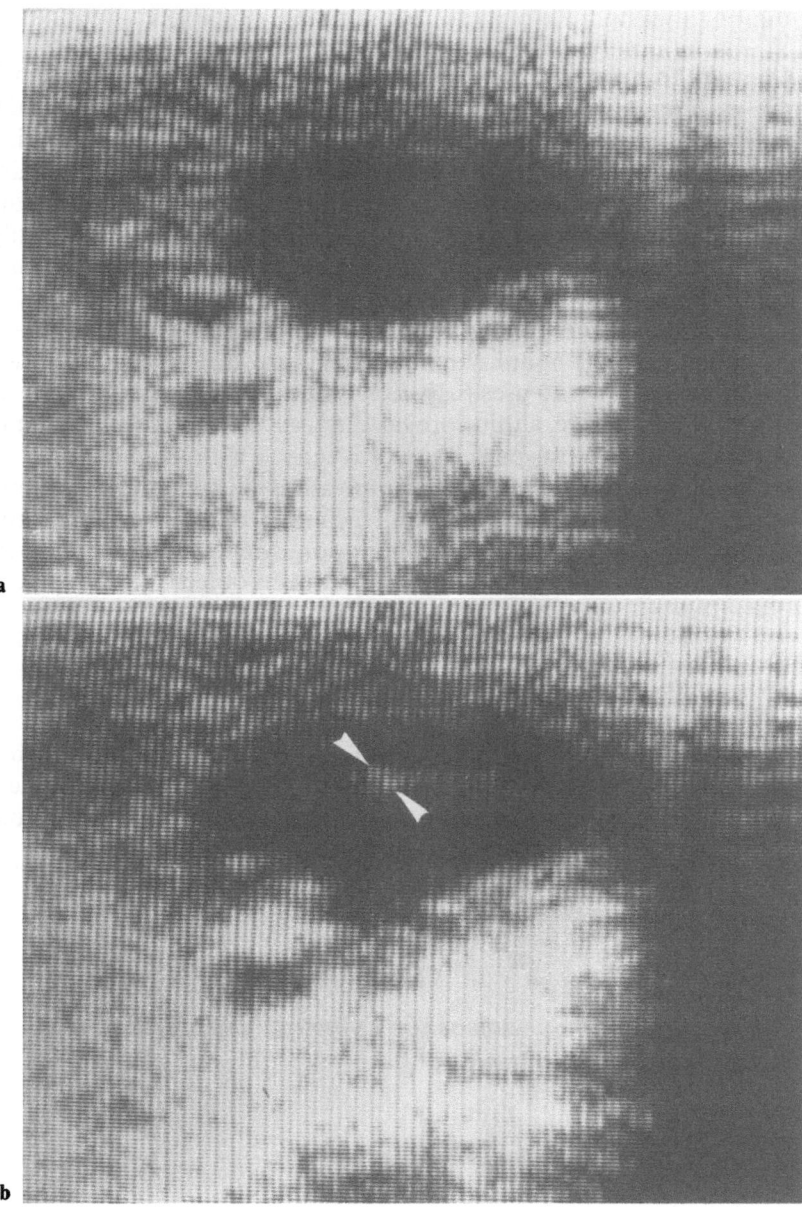

a

b

Fig. 37 a,b. Recurrence of a cervical tumor. **a** Recurrent tumor with area of central degeneration. **b** A fine needle has been inserted into the centrally degenerate tumor. No evidence of abscess is seen. The needle tip *(arrows)* is represented by a bright echo. This sonogram proves that needle tip visibility is obtainable even in relatively superficial tissues (the central cavity could not be reached by palpation alone, and initial cytologic findings were negative)

Breast

Contrary to many reports in the literature, sonography of the female breast is still used mainly to detect occult cysts in the radiodense breast and to evaluate palpable or mammographically visible nodules. While ultrasound is able to differentiate between cystic and solid masses, the malignancy or benignancy of a tumor still cannot be confidently established from sonographic features alone.

Although palpable masses corresponding to cysts are easily biopsied "blindly" and delineated by pneumocystography, there are rare instances where deep, indeterminate radiopacities in the mammogram will make ultrasound-guided aspiration desirable, especially if the lesion is nonpalpable.

Solid, palpable nodules in our patients are aspirated with a fan-like motion by the cytologist, who uses palpation to localize the mass. If the cytologic diagnosis is inconclusive, a thin core needle is used to obtain a histologic specimen.

Occasionally, a suspected tumor is missed with a blind biopsy. If there is a strong clinical or mammographic impression of carcinoma of the breast (cancer "feet," microcalcifications, etc.) and the results of initial cytologic investigations are negative, aspiration of the solid lesion is repeated under sonographic control. In two patients this enabled us to obtain objective confirmation of a suspected breast carcinoma.

Extremities

Most tumors of the extremities are discovered clinically and do not require ultrasound-guided biopsy. But if the tumor is very small or located near the bone, computed tomography or sonography can help to localize the lesion and guide the needle to it. Especially when cicatricial changes are present (e. g., after surgery or radiation therapy), biopsy under ultrasound guidance enables the prompt detection of a tumor recurrence.

3 Preparation of Specimens for Cytologic Examination — Possibilities and Limitations

G. PEDIO (pp. 68–79)

3.1 Introduction

The principal task of fine-needle biopsy within the context of ultrasonography and clinical diagnostics in general is the detection of malignant disease.

The technique of fine-needle aspiration biopsy can fulfill this task with great precision on the basis of the assessment of characteristic changes in individual cells.

The following prerequisites must be satisfied, however:

1. The aspirated specimen must be representative of the total lesion.
2. The aspirated cells must be kept in perfect condition.

Many laymen believe that malignant cells are monstrous in appearance, with grotesque nuclei and enormous nucleoles. In reality, it is not unusual for cancer cells to hide behind an innocent-looking facade. The cytologic diagnosis of malignancy is based on subtle alterations of nuclear structure. The preparation of material for cytologic evaluation aims at avoiding any artifactual cell changes caused by collection, smearing, and fixation of the specimen.

Three persons are crucial to the success of the examination:

1. The ultrasound specialist, who localizes the lesion, introduces the needle, and collects the specimen
2. The cytotechnologist, who smears, fixes, and stains the specimen
3. The cytologist, who is responsible for evaluating the specimen

Only well-coordinated teamwork among these experts can ensure an optimum result.

A continuous dialog should be maintained between the ultrasound specialist and the cytologist. Ideally, the two departments should be in close proximity to each other. The sonographer provides the cytologist with information on the patient's history, his clinical data, the precise location of the lesion aspirated, and the sonographic diagnosis. The cytologist, in turn, advises the ultrasound specialist on technical problems relating to collection of the specimen and, if possible, makes available trained personnel to prepare the specimen for examination.

Today cytologists can employ a special technique that allows a cell sample to be evaluated within minutes. This procedure is recommended for virtually every ultrasound-guided aspiration biopsy, as it permits a rapid assessment of the quality and adequacy of the specimen and provides an early tentative diagnosis. If the specimen is inadequate or a discrepancy is noted between cytologic and sonographic findings, a second aspiration may then be performed. There is no question but that this procedure leads to improved diagnostic results.

3.2 Collection and Processing of Cytologic Material

General Remarks

A suitable person (X-ray assistant, cytotechnologist, nurse) trained in the technique of preparing and fixing cytologic smears should assist the sonographer during the biopsy. Before the biopsy is performed, several glass slides and a cuvet of fixative solution should be placed on a side table. To avoid possible confusion, the patient's name should be written in pencil on the frosted end of the slide before the procedure is begun.

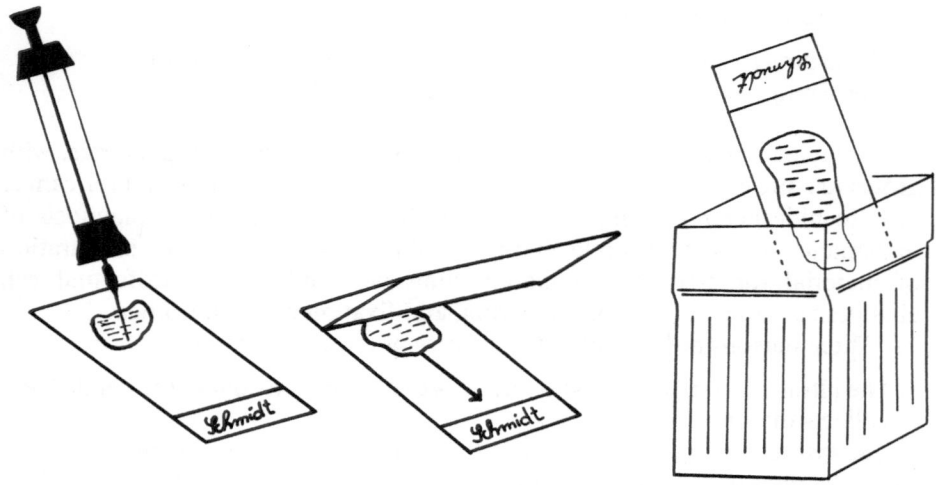

Fine-needle puncture

Fig. 38. Preparation and fixation of the smear

Procedure on Collection of Fluid Material

The fluid should be sent to the cytology laboratory in an untreated condition or with a few drops of hydromerphene added.

If an inflammatory process is suspected and sufficient material has been collected, a small amount of the aspirate should be stored under sterile conditions and submitted to a bacteriologic institute for microbiologic evaluation.

Procedure on Collection of Solid or Semisolid Material

Making the Smear. The solid or semisolid material is expelled onto one end of a glass slide. A second slide is then used to compress the specimen gently and spread it across the first slide (see Fig. 38).

Fixation. An accurate cytologic diagnosis depends less on the number of cells obtained than on their correct fixation. The type of fixation used will depend on the selected staining method. Two stains are principally used for tumor diagnosis: the May-Grünwald-Giemsa stain and the Papanicolaou stain. Fixation for Giemsa staining is done by air-drying the specimen, while smears must be wet-fixed for Papanicolaou staining. Before a smear is dried, it is best to immerse and fix it in Delaunay solution.

Delaunay solution: Absolute alcohol, 500 ml Acetone, 500 ml Trichloroacetic acid, 10–15 drops (1 mol/l)

Fixation time:For Papanicolaou rapid stain: 30s. For regular Papanicolaou stain: 30min or longer. Afterward the smear is air-dried and packaged in cardboard, plastic or Styrofoam.

70

Table 11. Staining methods

Purpose	Papanicolaou	Giemsa
Demonstration of nuclei	+ + +	+ +
Demonstration of cytoplasm	+	+ + +
Agreement with histologic sections	+ + +	+

+, fair; + +, good; + + +, excellent

Staining Procedure. All smears should be stained in a cytology laboratory. Either the Papanicolaou or Giemsa stain is satisfactory for tumor diagnosis. The advantages and disadvantages of each are listed in Table 11. The choice of staining method depends largely on the training and personal preference of the cytologist. As a rule, the Papanicolaou stain is used for general tumor diagnosis while the Giemsa method is preferred for hematologic cytology.

A very useful modification of the Papanicolaou method is the rapid stain. This technique allows cytologic material to be evaluated in about 7–10 min. The main advantage of this method is that if the specimen is found to be nonrepresentative, a second specimen can be aspirated at the same sitting. This reduces the rate of false-negative diagnoses.

Rapid stain by the Papanicolaou method

Fix in Delaunay solution	30 s
Rinse in 100% alcohol	
Rinse in 96% alcohol	
Rinse in 80% alcohol	
Rinse in 70% alcohol	
Rinse in 50% alcohol	
Rinse in distilled water	
Stain in hematoxylin	3 min
Rinse quickly in water	
Differentiate in 0.5% HCl	*very quickly*
Rinse in tepid water	3 min
Rinse in distilled water	
Rinse in 50% alcohol	
Rinse in 70% alcohol	
Rinse in 80% alcohol	
Rinse in 96% alcohol	
Stain in orange G-6	10 dips
Rinse twice in 96% alcohol	
Stain in EA 36	10 dips
Rinse in 96% alcohol	
Rinse twice in	100% alcohol
Rinse twice in xylene	
Mount in Eukitt	

Note: If sufficient material is available, it is recommended that several additional air-dried smears be prepared and left unstained. In selected cases these may be used later for special staining procedures (PAS, Congo red, Sudan black, DOPA).

3.3 Importance of Ultrasound-Guided Biopsy for Cytology

Rarely have two different techniques complemented each other so perfectly and led jointly to such outstanding diagnostic results as sonography and cytology. The ultrasound examination itself can uncover small, suspicious masses in the deepest organs, but without aspiration cytology it cannot give definitive information on the fine structure of the lesion or identify it as benign or malignant.

At the same time, the introduction of fine-needle aspiration biopsy under real-time ultrasound guidance has done much to expand the capabilities of diagnostic cytology. Body regions such as the pancreas, kidney, retroperitoneum, liver, and ovary, whose cytologies have been little explored, are now accessible to the cytologic method and can be selectively examined without surgical intervention.

As stated earlier, the main value of the combined ultrasound/cytology method is in the detection of malignant growths. Under optimum conditions the method may be expected to yield a positive, definitive diagnosis in 80%-90% of patients with malignant disease. In benign tumors, certain stages of inflammatory disease, and degenerative diseases, a cytologic diagnosis is considerably more difficult, if not impossible, to obtain.

In many cases the cytologic diagnosis will concur with the histologic diagnosis. The possibilities and limitations of the two methods are different, however (Table 12). The general advantages and limitations of fine-needle aspiration biopsy, which are briefly discussed below, are summarized in Table 13.

1. *High Diagnostic Accuracy*

Under the ideal conditions mentioned above, the selective aspiration of a malignant neoplasm will yield a definitive diagnosis in approximately 80%-90% of cases. As a rule, the cytologic diagnosis of a malignant process is highly reliable. The failure rate should not exceed 0.1%.

2, 3. *Simplicity of Technique and Rapidity of Diagnosis*

The aspiration technique is simple, is completed in a matter of seconds, is generally painless, leaves no scars, and may be done on an outpatient basis. In our department the specimens are routinely processed after abbreviated Papanicolaou staining. In this way the ultrasound specialist and clinician can be furnished with a diagnosis within 15-20 min. The advantages of this rapid diagnosis are obvious.

72

Table 12. Main differences between histology and cytology

Aspect	Histology	Cytology
Nature of specimen	Tissue	Cells
Diagnostic spectrum	All pathology	Neoplasia (chiefly)
Specimen collection	Operation (incision)	Aspiration biopsy
Costs	Significant	Very low
Time expenditure	Significant	Minimal

Table 13. Advantages and limitations of fine-needle aspiration biopsy

Advantages	Limitations
High diagnostic accuracy	Only masses beyond a certain size can be biopsied
Simple technique	False-negative results are unavoidable
Rapid diagnosis	Has limited value in the diagnosis of benign conditions
Reduction of patient anxiety	Cannot diagnose degenerative diseases
Low cost	
No contraindications	

4. *Alleviation of Patient Anxiety*

The patient, who suffers from the uncertainty of the pending diagnosis, can be told the nature of his disease right away. The clinician (or surgeon) can carefully plan further treatment. If a simple cyst is detected and emptied during the aspiration, this will not only provide a rapid diagnosis but will also have significant therapeutic value and relieve patient anxiety.

5. *Low Cost*

A fine-needle aspiration biopsy (specimen collection, processing, and evaluation) costs approximately 60 Swiss francs. There are no expenses relating to

operating room
surgical intervention
histologic processing
hospitalization.

6. *Complications and Contraindications*

Although the needle may penetrate several organs and blood vessels on the way to the area of interest, reports of immediate complications (hemorrhage, infection, etc.) are exceedingly rare [1].

The problem of tumor dissemination by the needle biopsy of a malignant lesion has frequently been discussed. While it is known that surgical procedures can cause the spread of cancer cells [32], this complication is rare with fine-nee-

Table 14. Local tumor dissemination after fine-needle aspiration biopsy

Tumor	No. of patients biopsied	Length of follow-up (years)	Local tumor dissemination	Reference
Pleomorphic adenoma of parotid gland	157	10	0	[32]
Carcinoma of prostate	469	3	0	[32]
Lymph node metastases	656	5	0	[33]

Table 15. Vascular tumor dissemination after fine-needle aspiration biopsy

Tumor	No. of patients biopsied/followed up	Length of follow-up (years)	Difference in survival time	Reference
Renal carcinoma	77/ 73	5	None	[167]
Breast carcinoma	370/370	15	None	[9]
Breast carcinoma	547/ 52	5	None	[9]

dle biopsies. In the cases described to date, either a relatively large-bore needle (e.g., Silverman needle) was used for the biopsy, or the caliber of the biopsy needle was not specified. Despite worldwide use of the method, there exists at present only one well-documented report of local tumor implantation after the repeated aspiration of a pancreatic carcinoma [39]. Follow-up studies in large patient series confirm the fundamental safety of fine-needle aspiration biopsy (Tables 14 and 15).

7. *Limitations of the Method*

The Limitations of the method are listed in Table 13.

a) As a rule, tumor nodules must reach a certain size before percutaneous aspiration is feasible. This means that aspiration biopsy can practically never furnish an early diagnosis of cancer.

b) Despite flawless technique, it must be acknowledged that a certain percentage of malignant tumors will not be detected. For example, the needle may miss the tumor completely, or heavily fibrotic tissue may prevent the aspiration of malignant cells. The rate of false-negative diagnoses is approximately 5%-10%.

It must be emphasized again that in the face of persistent clinical suspicion or obscure findings negative cytologioc results do not obviate the need for histologic investigation.

c) Cytology is of limited value in classifying benign tumors or benign processes. This is because a benign tissue change often does not exhibit a characteristic cell type. Cytologic diagnosis must be based on a peculiar arrangement or proliferation of normal cells.

74

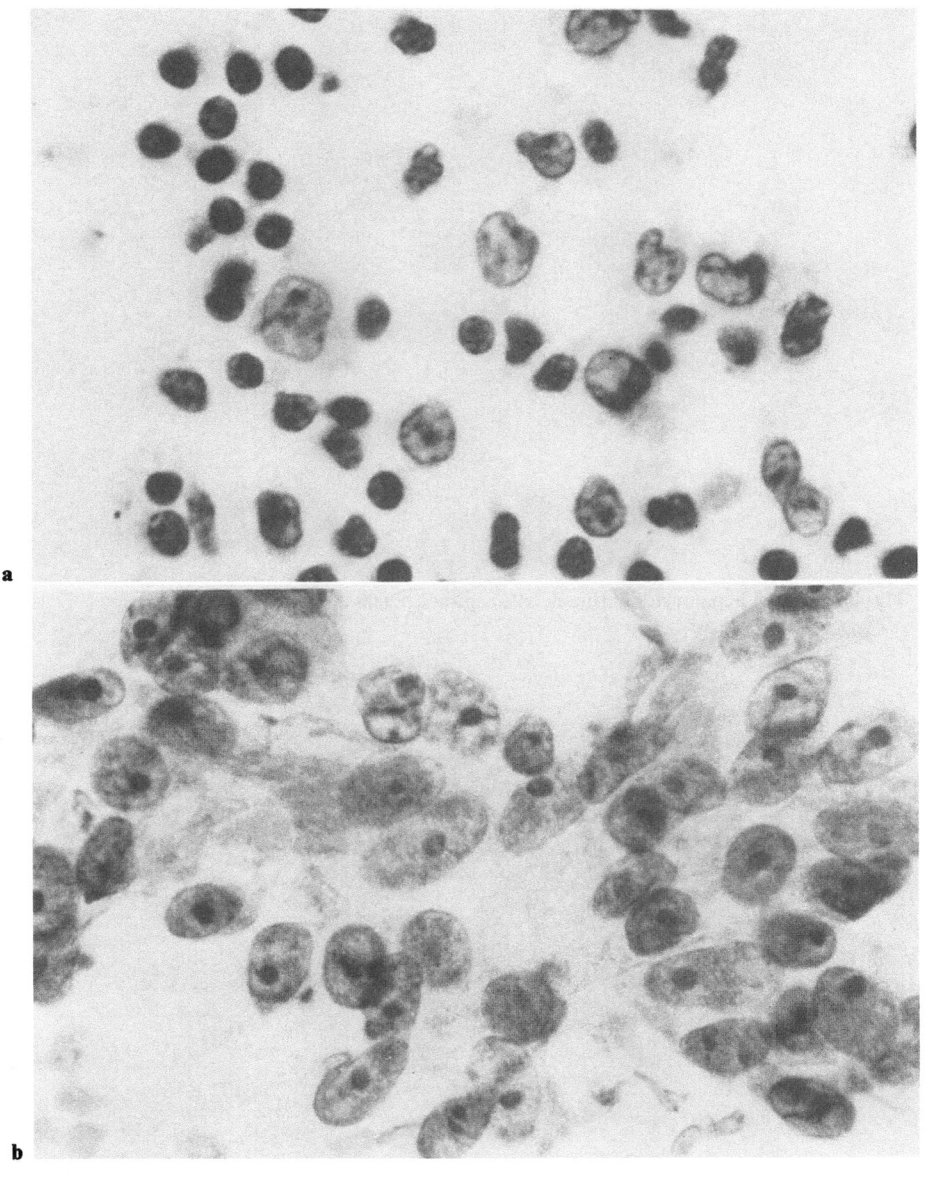

Fig. 39a,b. Fine-needle aspirate from a pancreatic carcinoma. **a** Typical malignant cell cluster. **b** Higher-power view of malignant cell cluster. × 600

75

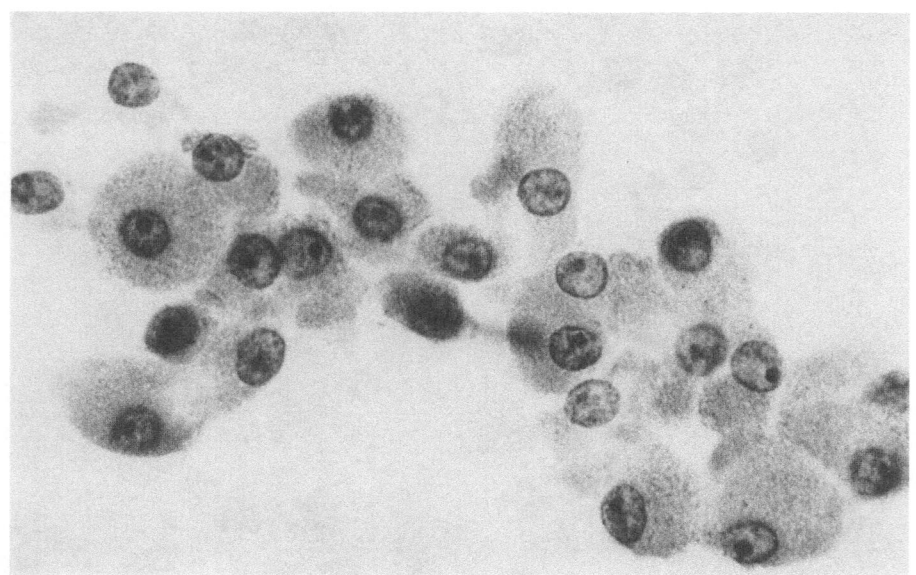

Fig. 40. Normal hepatocytes in fine-needle aspirate. × 600

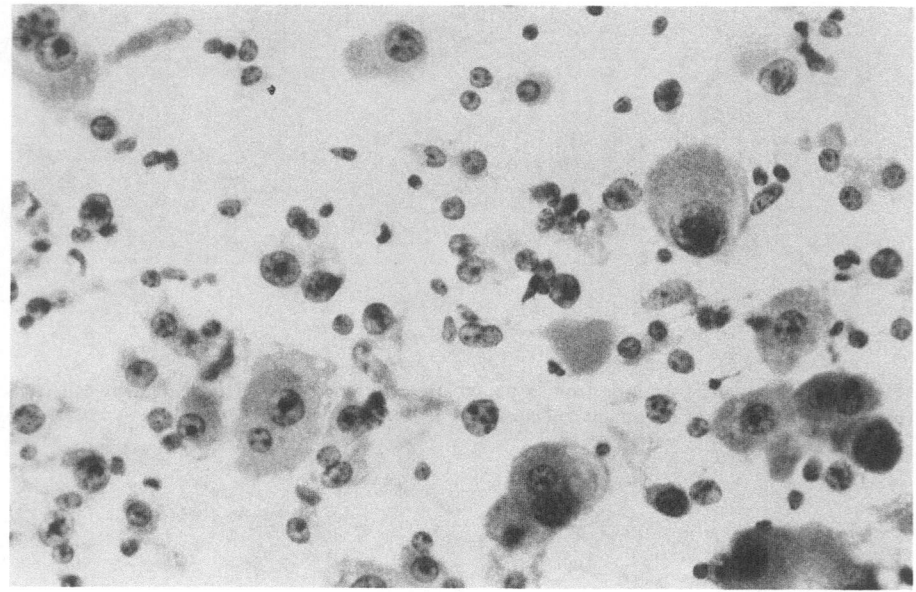

Fig. 41. Hepatoma, scattered malignant cells in fine-needle aspirate. × 400

Fulminating inflammatory processes are easily recognized in cytologic smears. In fibrosed forms, however, aspiration probably will not be rewarding.

Degenerative diseases (cirrhosis, atherosclerosis, etc.) are not amenable to cytologic diagnosis.

3.4 Principal Applications of Ultrasound-Guided Fine-Needle Biopsy

Ultrasound-guided fine-needle aspiration biopsy is most frequently used to investigate suspected tumors of the abdominal cavity. The capabilities and limitations of the cytologic method are briefly stated below for each organ:

1. *Pancreas:* Outstanding results in the diagnosis of pancreatic carcinomas (Fig. 39 a,b) and benign cystic masses. Good results in the diagnosis of fulminating inflammations. Fibrosis of the pancreas cannot be diagnosed.
2. *Liver:* Outstanding results in the detection of metastatic growths. Often the method can provide informationon the nature of the primary tumor (Fig. 40 shows normal liver cells). Very good results are obtained in primary hepatic carcinomas (Fig. 41) and carcinoids. With hydatid cysts, it is possible to demonstrate the causativeorganism or parts of it. Detection of hepatic adenoma is difficult. The finding of a hemangioma is nonspecific. In both these cases the absence of malignant cells is the only report that can be given.
   In hepatitis and hepatic cirrhosis, the method provides minimal information on the nature of the disease.
3. *Retroperitoneum:* Results are very good in malignant lymphomas (Fig. 42 a,b), carcinomas, and sarcomas, though sarcomas are difficult to classify as to type. Retroperitoneal fibrosis (Ormond's disease) is difficult to diagnose.
4. *Kidney and Adrenal:* Excellent results are recorded in the diagnosis of carcinoma of the kidney and renal pelvis (Fig. 43). Recently, good results have been reported in the evaluation of renal transplants. Results are also good in adrenal carcinoma, although it can be very difficult to distinguish between a primary tumor and metastatic involvement.
   Myelolipoma is readily diagnosed. Adenomas of the kidneys and adrenals are difficult to identify.
5. *Ovary:* Generally, ovarian carcinoma is easy to diagnose. So far little study has been done on the classifiation of ovarian neoplasms into different histologic subgroups.

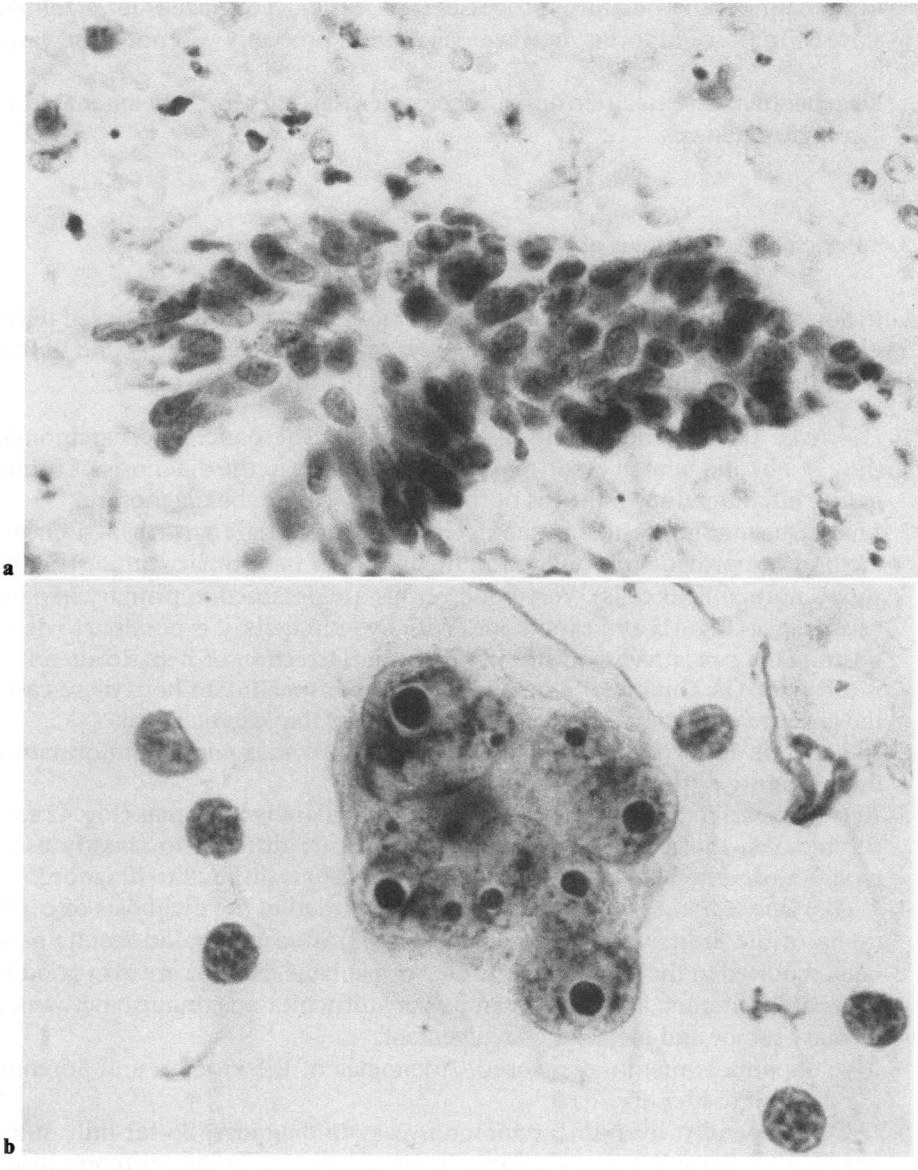

Fig. 42 a,b. Fine-needle aspirate. **a** Malignant non-Hodgkin's lymphoma of the centroblastic/centrocytic type. **b** Hodgkin's disease, Sternberg-Reed cells. × 800

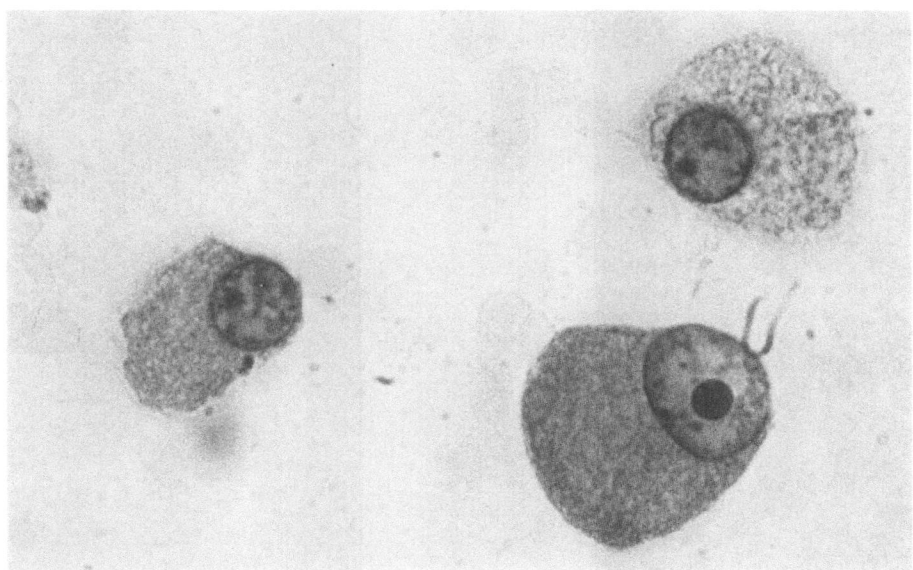

Fig. 43. Fine-needle aspirate. Classic hypernephroma cells. × 1200

4 Biopsy for Histologic Examination

4.1 Core Biopsy

Fine needles for the aspiration of cytologic material from soft tissues are distinguished by their small external diameter, which is less than 1 mm and is usually between 0.6 and 0.8 mm. These needles require a relatively strong aspiration to collect an adequate sample of cellular material. There are situations in which the aspiration of cytologic material fails to establish a diagnosis, and a histologic examination is necessary. For example, in the case of a malignant lymphoma it can be very difficult to identify Hodgkin's cells in a cytologic smear, and a hepatoma frequently cannot be diagnosed. Of course, there are other neoplastic disorders in which even the removal of a large specimen for histologic study will in itself fail to disclose the nature of the disease.

In some cases a histologic examination may be indicated because a well-equipped cytology laboratory is not available.

Various biopsy needles may be used to obtain material for histologic examination. All operate by excising a core of tissue whose histologic features are then analyzed. Aspiration either is not used at all, as in the Tru-Cut needle, or else it is subordinate to the cutting action of the needle.

Every operator familiar with fine-needle aspiration biopsies knows that the amount of tissue collected is critically influenced by the amount of suction ap-

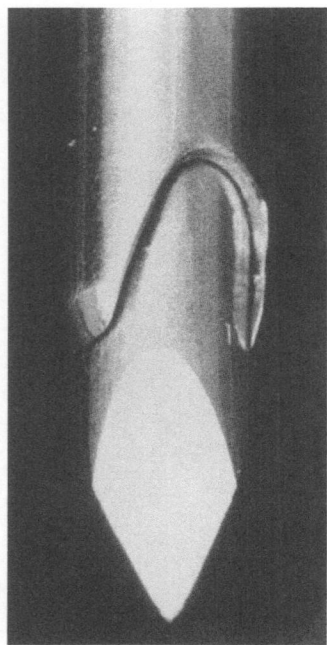 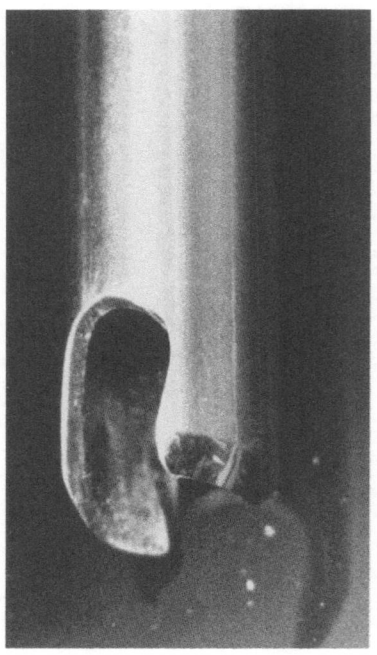

Fig. 44. Thin cutting-edge needle. The stylet is advanced for insertion through the skin

Fig. 45. Thin cutting-edge needle. The stylet is retracted, exposing the cutting edges and lumen for the reception of tissue

plied. Also, ultrasound monitoring has confirmed that elastic soft-tissue organs can be pushed aside rather than penetrated by even a sharp aspiration needle. This occasionally leads to problems in aspirations of the liver [153].

4.2 The Thin Cutting-Edge Needle

Prompted by these drawbacks of aspiration biopsies, we developed a thin cutting-edge needle (or fine core needle) whose external diameter is equal to or only slightly larger than that of the standard aspiration needle. The thin cutting-edge needle is armed with a pointed stylet for insertion. After reaching the area of interest, the stylet is withdrawn, and continuous (and variable) negative pressure is applied through the lumen, thereby attaching the needle tip to the tissue by suction. With the stylet removed, the needle tip presents two diametrically opposed cutting edges separated by deep notches (Figs. 44 and 45). Despite its thinness, the needle is capable of excising and retrieving a cylindrical core of tissue that is adequate for histologic evaluation. Clockwise rotation of the needle may assist the cutting process but is not mandatory. The thin cutting-edge needles are available in various calibers (see Table 2). Figure 46 shows the nee-

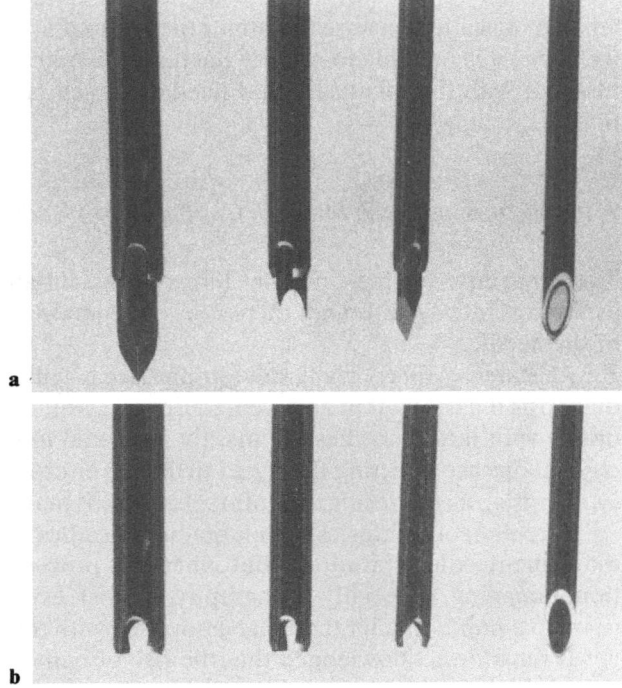

Fig. 46a,b. The different calibers of the thin cutting-edge needle. **a** Ready for skin insertion with stylet advanced. The standard Chiba fine needle *(far right)* is shown for comparison. **b** Ready for tissue sampling with stylet retracted

dles in comparison with the Chiba needle, first with stylets in place for insertion through the skin (Fig. 46a) and then with stylets removed for obtaining the specimen (Fig. 46b).

The use of a pointed stylet overcomes the problem of organ-capsule elasticity and also makes it easier to take biopsies within parenchymatous organs, which are compartmentalized by numerous elastic elements (septa, vessels).

The presence of the stylet during insertion stiffens the thin needle and makes it easier to direct. In addition, the stylet only pierces the capsule of the target organ without cutting out tissue, as occurs with ordinary cutting needles. This reduces the risk of hemorrhage.

Basically the thin cutting-edge needle represents a combination of the fine aspiration needle and conventional core needle. It was designed chiefly for the atraumatic retrieval of specimens that would allow a histologic evaluation of diffuse hepatic or renal parenchymal disease. Additionally, we have found that the thin cutting-edge needle is superior to ordinary fine needles in biopsies of very firm tumors or scar tissue and is useful in the evaluation of suspected malignant lymphoma. It has also been used in palpable masses of the breast and thyroid, in which cases sonographic guidance is usually unnecessary.

Another application is in the diagnosis of certain skeletal tumors, especially when metastatic. Because the tumor tissue often invades soft tissues adjacent to the bone, it is possible to classify the tumor by retrieving a core of juxtaosseous material with the relatively rigid needle. Sometimes this will obviate the need for a bone biopsy.

Principle of Biopsy with the Thin Cutting-Edge Needle

The procedure for the fine core biopsy is essentially the same as that for the aspiration biopsy, although there are some notable differences in the handling of the needle.

As stated earlier, core tissue samples are usually unnecessary for oncologic diagnosis if a competent and well-equipped cytology laboratory is available. Biopsies with larger needles are mainly indicated in cases of generalized parenchymal disease affecting the liver (cirrhosis) or especially the kidney (glomerulonephritis), as the result will influence patient management.

Percutaneous biopsies with large-bore needles are inherently more invasive than fine-needle aspirations. But when the procedure is guided by cross-sectional imaging, especially sonography, the risk even with larger-gauge needles is, up to a point, smaller than that associated with traditional blind punctures.

It must be acknowledged that the risk of hemorrhage and other complications is higher with larger-caliber needles, some of which exert a tearing action on tissues. This fact prompted us to develop a new technique which enables histologic specimens to be taken with a relatively small-caliber needle at approximately the same risk associated with fine-needle aspirations. As before, the biopsy is performed under real-time ultrasound guidance with respiration suspended if possible.

Biopsies with the thin cutting-edge needle are more complex and time-consuming than biopsies with regular cutting needles, but we feel that the safety and reliability of the technique outweigh these disadvantages.

While the core of tissue retrieved with the thin needle has a very small diameter (less than 1 mm), the length of the specimen is considerable (1–3 cm) and should enable the pathologist to draw valid conclusions on the histologic structure of the excised tissue.

The instrument setup for biopsies with the thin cutting-edge needle is analogous to that for fine-needle aspirations, except that a somewhat larger needle guide is used (we use a plastic, conical guide suitable for all biopsy needles and drainage tubes), as well as a locking vacuum syringe. The fenestrated towel for draping the prepared skin and the plastic bag for sterile packaging of the transducer are the same as those used for fine-needle aspirations (Fig. 47). When the thinnest cutting-edge needle is used (0.78 mm), all other equipment is identical to that in fine-needle aspirations because the needle calibers are virtually identical. The particular caliber that is selected will depend on the nature of the investigation and the organ to be biopsied.

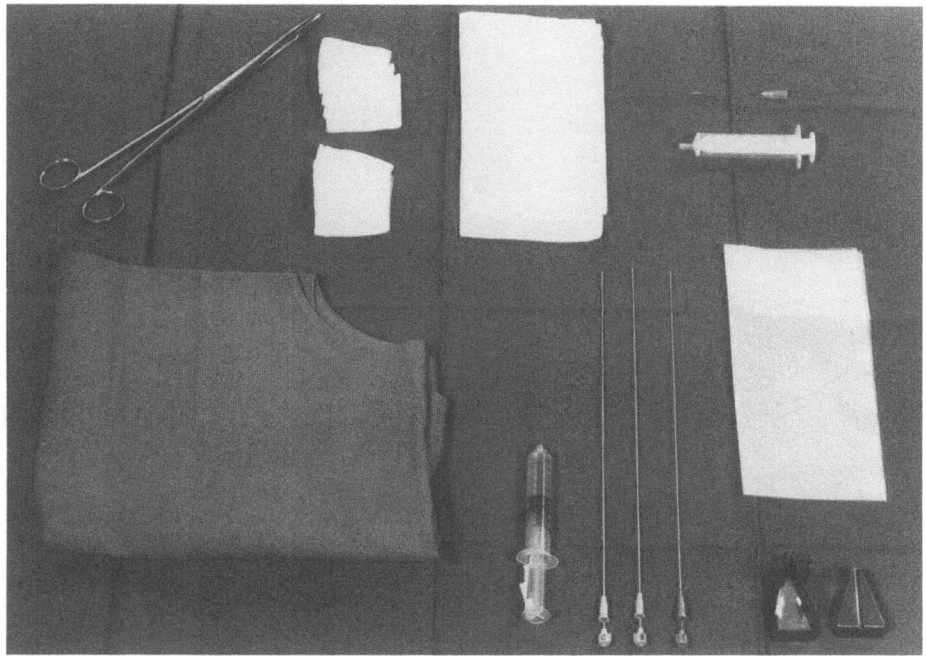

Fig. 47. Instrument setup for biopsy with the thin cutting-edge needle. Needles of all three calibers have been laid out, but in other respects the setup is like that of a fine-needle aspiration. Local anesthesia is necessary only when the larger calibers (0.95 mm and 1.2 mm) are employed

Recently the thin cutting-edge needle has been used to good advantage in evaluations of certain focal diseases, owing particularly to the very low risk that exists when the smallest needle caliber is used. The range of indications for biopsies with the fine-core needle is presented below.

Indications for Biopsy with the Thin Cutting-Edge Needle

1. Diffuse diseases of the parenchymatous organs
   Liver (cirrhosis, hepatitis)
   Kidney (glomerulonephritis)
2. Focal diseases of the parenchymatous organs
   a) Under ultrasound or computed tomographic guidance:
      Unavailability of cytology laboratory
      Inconclusiveness of cytologic evaluation
      Centrally necrotic tumors
      Richly vascular tumors that yield excessive blood on aspiration with a fine needle
      Tumors with a strong fibrotic component (e.g., sclerosing form of Hodgkin's disease, certain intestinal growths), scar tissue

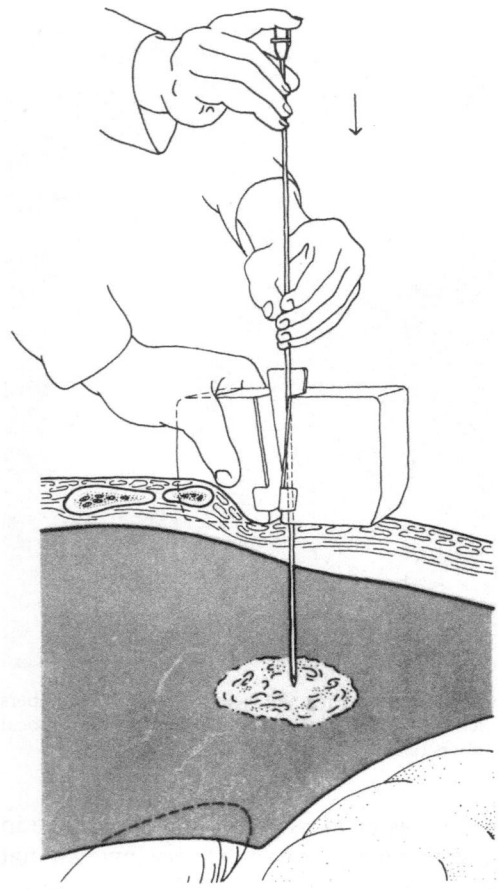

Fig. 48. The cutting-edge needle with indwelling stylet is inserted in to the periphery of the focal anomaly (with diffuse disease it is advanced to a point just below or just outside the capsule)

Skeletal tumors with invasion of juxtaosseous soft tissues
Need to grade malignant lymphomas
Intrathoracic tumors.
b) Guided by direct palpation, without ultrasound:
Solid breast nodules
Thyroid nodules (cytology often unclear)
Superficial soft-tissue nodules
Firm lymph node metastases (e. g., in cervical region)
Prostatic biopsy.

The decision whether to use a fine aspiration needle or our thin cutting-edge needle will also depend on available pathology facilities. If a cytologist is not immediately available, then the main advantage of fine-needle aspiration, rapid evaluation, is lost. In this case it is better to rely on histologic findings. Of

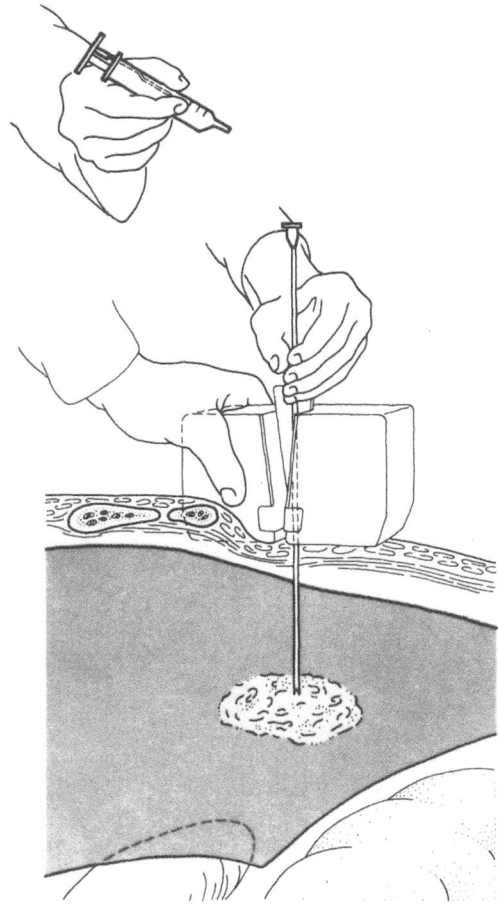

Fig. 49. The stylet is removed and the
locking vacuum syringe is mounted

course, the pathologist should be notified that he will be handling small tissue
samples that require special processing.

Biopsy with the thin cutting-edge needle is performed in steps. Following
prebiopsy evaluation, the target organ is localized with the apertured transducer, and the stylet-armed needle is introduced through the skin and into the subcutaneous fatty tissue, or it may be advanced directly through the organ capsule
or into the periphery of a focal lesion (Fig. 48).

After the stylet is removed, a special 10-ml plastic syringe is connected to
the needle hub (Fig. 49). A locking mechanism on the syringe plunger makes it
possible to lock the plunger in a position that will maintain a vacuum of 3–5 ml,
provided the needle tip does not enter a large blood vessel or cyst (Fig. 50). Now
the needle is thrust 1–3 cm (depending on findings) into the area of interest
(Fig. 51). If desired, the needle may be rotated clockwise from one-half to one
turn as the organ is entered, but this is not essential. When the specimen has

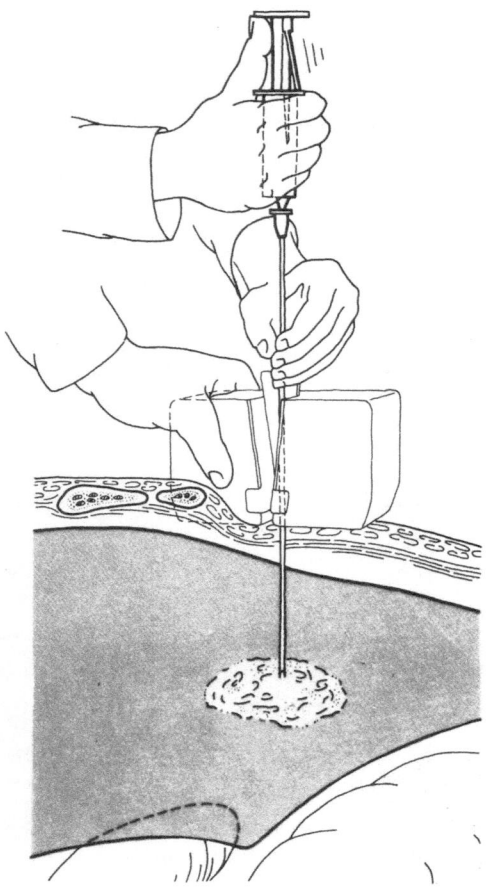

Fig. 50. The plunger of the vacuum syringe is drawn back and locked to create a maximum of 5 ml suction. The needle is now ready for tissue retrieval

been excised, the suction in the syringe will draw it into the lumen of the needle. We perform this maneuver two or three times, i.e., withdraw the needle to its starting point under sonographic vision and then readvance it with a brisk jabbing motion. If the puncture is made too slowly, there will be a tendency for the elastic tissue to be pushed aside by the needle, which may not retrieve enough material for histologic processing.

Practice in tissue preparations (liver, kidney, etc.) will make it easier to grasp the correct use of this instrument and is highly recommended. In very firm tissue (fibrotic tumor tissue, certain intestinal tumors, wide areas of fibrosis, breast nodules, kidneys), a stronger suction will have to be applied (up to 5 ml of vacuum); less suction is needed in softer, more vascular organs and tumors. The suction can be adjusted as needed with the aid of the locking syringe.

Strong suction carries a greater risk of aspirating blood along with the tissue core. As this can be difficult to predict, we flush the syringe and needle beforehand with saline to which a small amount of Liquaemin has been added (ap-

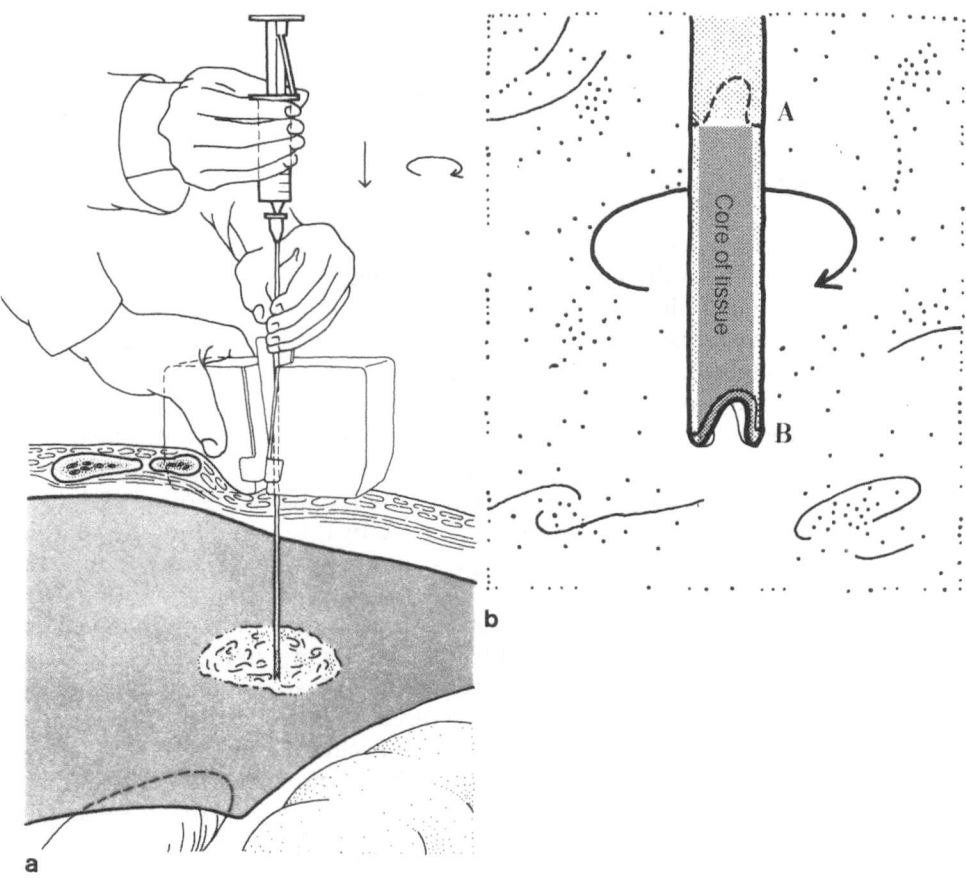

Fig. 51 a,b. Taking the specimen. **a** The physician thrusts the needle 1–3 cm into the lesion or organ *(straight arrow)*, while rotating it slightly in a clockwise direction *(curved arrow)*. **b** Detail of the needle tip during tissue removal: initial position *(A)* and final position *(B)* after excision of the specimen, which is now in the distal portion of the needle. In addition to the vertical "punch" movement, the needle can be simultaneously rotated in a clockwise direction *(arrow)*, corresponding to the grind of the cutting edge, to help excise the specimen

prox. 1 drop Liquaemin to 20 ml physiologic NaCl). The core of tissue is easily identified in the unclotted blood.

Before the needle is withdrawn, the plunger is generally released to ensure that the tissue core remains in the needle. If the specimen is drawn into the syringe, however, it is easily flushed out, and this may even be a safer retrieval technique. Further processing of the tissue is done in the pathology laboratory and must allow for the very small size of the specimen.

At present we are working on an automatic device for use with the thin cutting-edge needle (Angiomed, D-7505 Ettlingen) that will enable specimens to be taken in seconds even from deeply situated organs. Clinical testing of this device is not yet complete.

5 A Pathologist's View of Needle Biopsy

H. R. Burger (pp. 88–95)

5.1 Introduction

Histopathologic diagnosis still occupies a central place in the investigation of many diseases. With the introduction of new techniques of biopsy and tissue sampling, histopathology has grown in status from an ancillary study in post-mortem examinations to a crucial investigation in live patients. Increasing reliance has been placed on the assumption that a small sample can indeed be representative of an entire organ or of the entire lesion.

Because every biopsy carries some degree of risk, the physician active in diagnosis will seek to limit the scale of the procedure as much as possible in order to minimize the risk. The result is a tendency toward the taking of smaller specimens. At the same time, this tendency is limited by the demands of the pathologist, who requires an adequate and representative sample in order to make an evaluation.

Today cytology is making an important contribution to morphological diagnosis. It has become an indispensable tool, particularly in the classification of tumors. Even so, it is still necessary to rely on histologic examination in the diagnosis of many generalized parenchymal diseases, in which an appreciation of the intact tissue structure is necessary for an accurate evaluation. In the past, histologic specimens from organs not accessible to direct incision or endoscopy could be obtained only by the use of biopsy needles that carried a substantial risk of trauma. The advantage of the thin cutting-edge needle is that it greatly reduces traumatic risk while still providing adequate material for histologic processing and evaluation.

5.2 Methods of Histologic Processing

Like all biopsy procedures, thin-needle core biopsies require close cooperation between the pathologist and the physician performing the biopsy. This is necessary to achieve the high diagnostic yield that will justify the risk of the biopsy. Because the morphological methodology can vary a great deal depending on the nature of the clinical problem, a preliminary consultation is strongly advised especially when using biopsy methods that furnish a minimal amount of material. If the physician managing the investigation is someone other than the examiner, it is advised that the pathologist also consult with the clinician, who is generally not present at the biopsy.

We use two methods to ensure that specimens are processed in the freshest condition possible. One method is to have the specimen received by the technical assistant present at the biopsy. The assistant must know how to handle the

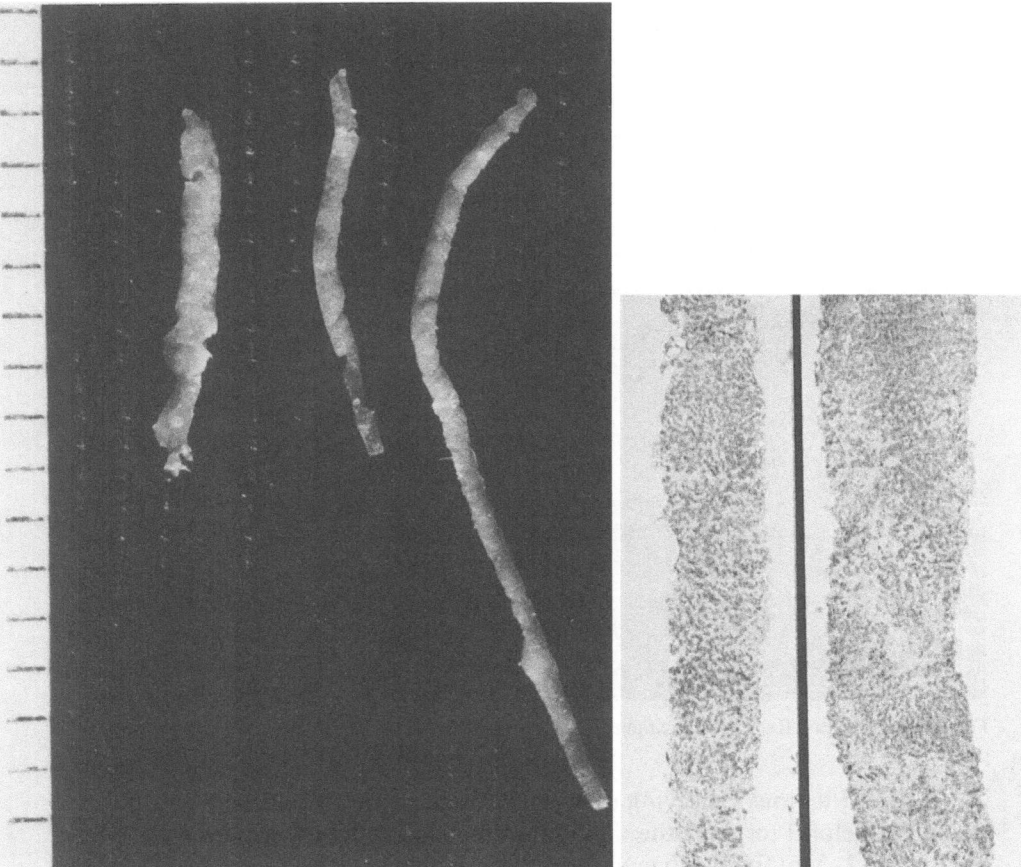

b

Fig. 52 a,b. Biopsy material. **a** Comparison of a conventional core biopsy and a fine core biopsy. Gross appearance of core specimens taken from the liver (*scale* in millimeters). The shorter, thick core (*left half of picture*) was obtained with a Tru-Cut needle. **b** Comparison of fine core specimens from the liver obtained with thin cutting-edge needles (*left* needle diameter 0.95 mm; *right*, 1,2 mm)

material properly and how to place it into fixative without traumatizing it. This means that the technical staff of the diagnostic department has to be instructed in histopathologic processing and technique. In special cases such as renal biopsy or studies requiring complex preparation of the material, it has proved more expedient to send a histology laboratory assistant to the biopsy. The extra effort is justified by improved results.

The main problem with the fine core needle is getting the thin tissue core (Fig. 52 a) from the lumen of the needle into the fixative. This is facilitated by flushing the needle beforehand with heparin to prevent the clotting of aspirated blood. After the biopsy there is usually no difficulty in expelling the tissue core, although the specimen may occasionally fragment depending on its consistency (Fig. 53).

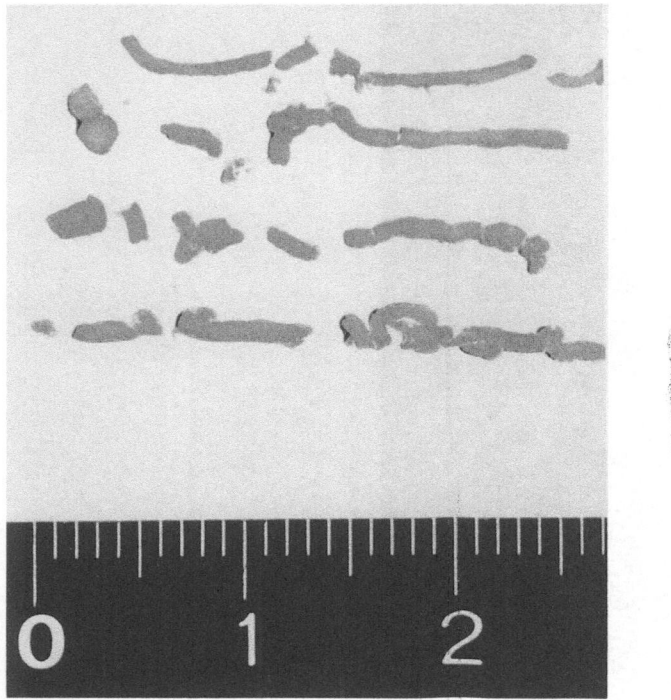

Fig. 53. Fragmented fine core specimens from a necrotic lesion with abscess (*scale* in centimeters)

To avoid tedious retrieving of small tissue particles from a large fluid volume, it is helpful to place the material into small, 5- to 10-ml specimen tubes containing 2–3 ml fixative (usually 4% formaldehyde). The contents of the tube are poured directly into a capsule (Tissuetek) lined with filter paper without touching the biopsy material with forceps or otherwise traumatizing it. Once in the capsule, which is available in several colors, the material can be further processed automatically until it is embedded in paraffin or another suitable medium.

If a large amount of blood is present, it can be difficult to locate the tissue in the specimen tube. In this case the syringe may be discharged into a petri dish, although this requires that the material subsequently be transferred to the fixative vessel with a forceps or pipette and thus exposes it to an additional source of trauma. This can be avoided by placing a Tissuetek capsule lined with filter paper into the petri dish and expelling the contents of the needle directly into the capsule. Material not wanted for further processing, such as clots, fibrin shreds, and blood, can be drawn off with a pipette. The sealed capsules, immersed in fixative and labeled, serve as containers for transport to the histopathology laboratory.

The material obtained with the thin needle can then be processed further in the same way as any other biopsy specimen. Depending on the type of fixative

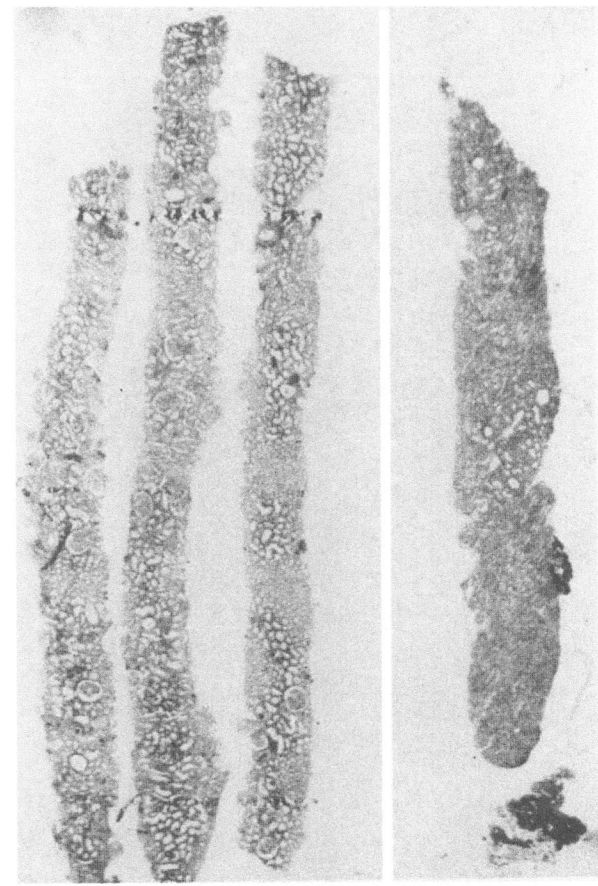

Fig. 54. Comparison of a conventional renal core specimen *(right)* and a specimen obtained with the thin cutting-edge needle *(left)* (core is in three parts). × 14

used, the specimen may be examined with the electron microscope or studied by immunohistochemical methods and techniques applied to frozen sections. An advantage of the thin cutting-edge needle is that, with proper technique, the length of the biopsy core is substantial. The thinness of the core relative to conventional biopsy needles does not lessen the diagnostic value of the specimen (Fig. 54).

5.3 Results

We have reviewed the specimens taken from the first 78 patients who underwent core biopsies with the thin cutting-edge needle. Initially a fine-needle aspiration for cytologic evaluation was concurrently performed in 39 of the pat-

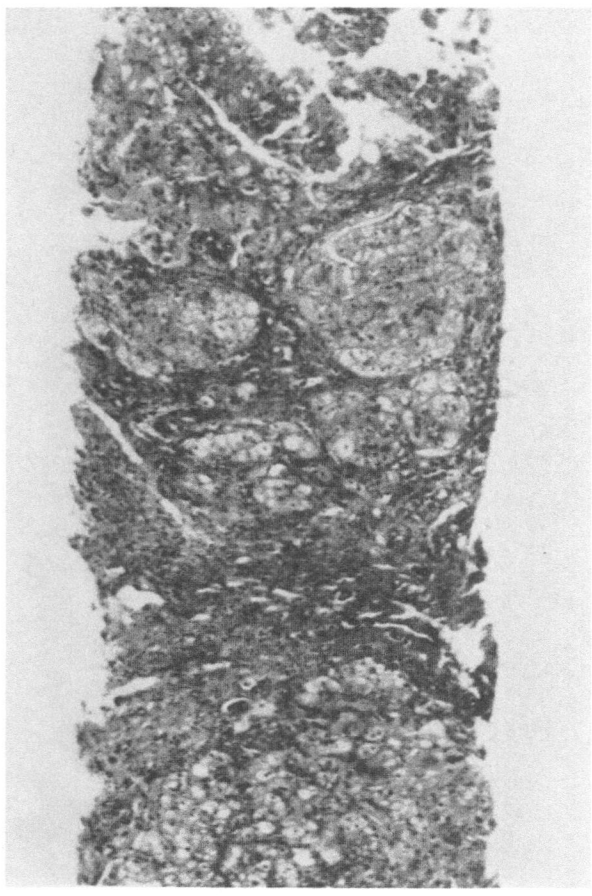

Fig. 55. Histologic section from a core obtained with the thin cutting-edge needle in hepatic cirrhosis. ×65

ients. Also during the introductory phase, 18 other patients were biopsied with a conventional needle of the Tru-Cut type.

In 20 of the 78 patients (25%), the fine core biopsy did not yield a positive result. Twelve of these 20 patients underwent a concurrent fine-needle aspiration, which was negative in six cases. In six other cases the cytologic result was positive. In three of the patients with negative cytology, the fine core biopsy was positive.

Most failures with the thin cutting-edge needle in the 20 cases mentioned above occurred because the needle withdrew insufficient representative material (perhaps only blood) while the excised tissue core remained within the organ. In firm tumors or in hepatic cirrhosis (Fig. 55), this can occur when the operator is too tentative in taking the biopsy. There was only one case where the specimen could not be evaluated for histotechnical reasons; it had become lost during processing due to the small size of the tissue particles. Finally, it should be noted that most failures with fine core biopsies occurred during the introducto-

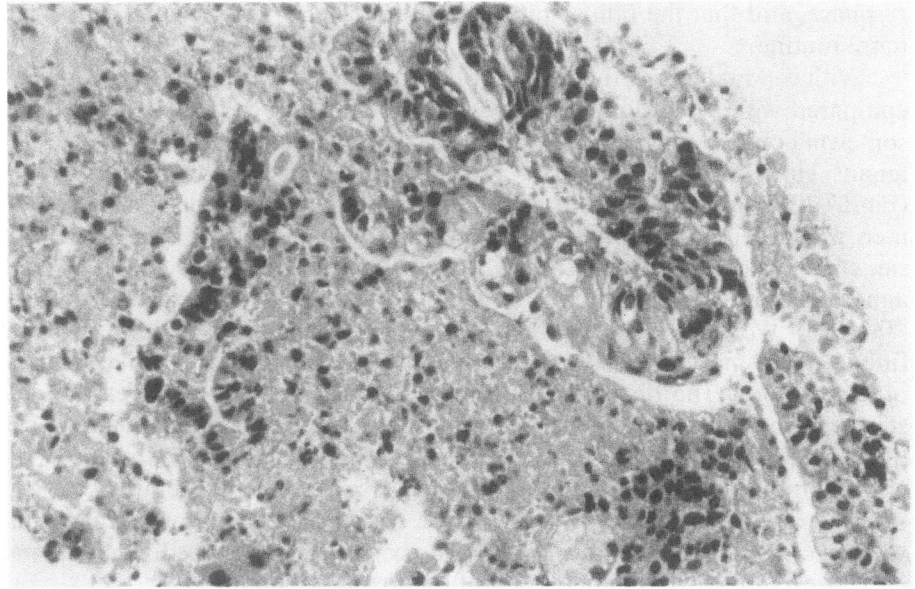

Fig. 56. High-power view of a fine-core liver biopsy: adenocarcinoma. The specimen was obtained with a thin cutting-edge needle. × 320

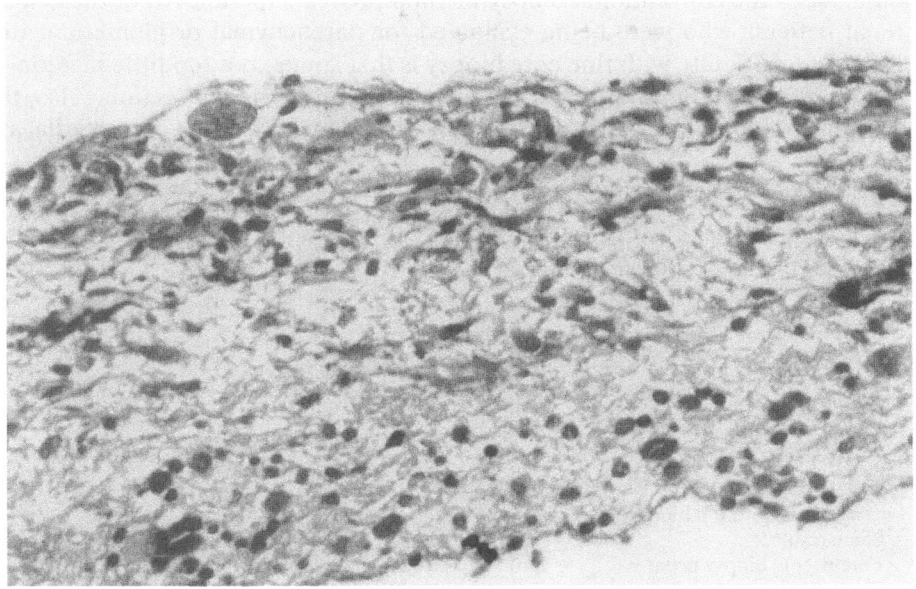

Fig. 57. High-power view of a core specimen from the retroperitoneum in confirmed Hodgkin's disease: Hodgkin's granuloma. The specimen was obtained with a thin cutting-edge needle. × 320

ry phase, and that the failure rate declined drastically as the method became more routine.

With certain tumors, the results of fine core biopsies are not very conclusive compared with aspiration cytology. Usually, the cutting-edge needle provides somewhat better accuracy in the diagnosis of hepatoma (Fig. 56). Its use in malignant Hodgkin's lymphoma is recommended only if the tumor is large (Fig. 57). When we look at the 39 cases in which a concurrent cytologic specimen was obtained, we find that the cytologic and histologic results were the same in 22 cases. In ten cases aspiration cytology was more accurate, i. e., its diagnostic information was more valuable. In seven cases the reverse was true (Table 16). We disregard cases in which the result could not be improved over fine-needle aspiration because of negative staining results or negative results of other methods. The diagnostic accuracy of fine core biopsy increased when staining properties, stromal features, vascular features, or similar characteristics of the tissue environment were available for assessment, or when the use of special techniques such as immunofluorescence, immunohistochemistry, or electron microscopy enabled the lesion to be characterized more accurately than with cytology. Most poor results with fine core biopsy occurred when the needle retrieved only soft tissue instead of the suspected tumor.

Conditions that are not amenable to cytodiagnosis, such as parenchymal diseases of the liver and kidney, can be investigated with the thin core needle. In the past, such diseases were investigated by the use of relatively large-bore needles to ensure an adequate tissue yield. This prompted us to compare the two methods in 18 patients. In eight cases the results were equivalent. In eight other cases the conventional biopsy method proved superior. All of these were renal patients who were being evaluated for parenchymal or glomerular disease. One difficulty with fine core biopsy is that sometimes too little material is left over for the immunofluorescent examination of a frozen section. Also, the sampling of cortical tissue is occasionally difficult with the fine core needle, ap-

Table 16. Fine core biopsy compared with conventional core biopsy and fine-needle aspiration biopsy

	n	(%)
Conventional core biopsy		
Same result	8	(44)
Conventional biopsy better	8	(44)
Fine core biopsy better	2	(44)
Total	18	(100)
Fine-needle aspiration biopsy		
Same result	22	(56)
Fine-needle biopsy better	10	(26)
Fine core biopsy better	7	(18)
Total	39	(100)

parently for reasons other than localization. On the other hand, our comparative series includes two cases in which fine core biopsy yielded by far the best result. Since these trials we have, in fact, abandoned all other renal biopsy methods in favor of the fine core technique, which we perform under real-time sonographic control. We have had no additional diagnostic failures.

Obviously, no qualitative difference may be expected in the diagnostic or histologic evaluation of the two biopsy methods. The difference is purely quantitative, and in this respect the fine core method proved entirely comparable to the conventional core biopsy. If it should be confirmed that use of the thin cutting-edge needle reduces the risk of biopsy procedure its use will also be fully justified from the standpoint of the morphologist.

6 Does Needle Biopsy Promote Tumor Spread?

The histologic examination is acknowledged as the most accurate and reliable method of establishing the nature of an autonomous growth and classifying it as benign or malignant. Today cytologic methods have attained a similarly high status. Despite the development of modern cross-sectional imaging methods, including nuclear magnetic resonance and digital subtraction angiography, the histologic examination still has a unique and important role in the investigation of suspicious tissue.

Following the gross morphologic detection of a tumor, it is necessary to establish a pathologic diagnosis, for different tumor types with similar clinical presentations may require radically different therapies or even no special therapy at all. The simplest way to do this is by performing a needle biopsy to obtain cytologic or histologic material. Accurate tumor staging is no longer conceivable without the direct microscopic analysis of specimens.

Since the development of percutaneous needle biopsy some 25 years ago, the method has repeatedly been characterized as dangerous, first because of the potential for organic injury and consequent *hemorrage,* and second because of the presumed danger of *tumor cell dissemination* and *metastasis.*

Traumatic organ lesions caused by needle biopsy and the related dangers are discussed in the chapters dealing with biopsies of specific organs. They depend on technical factors. The traumatic risk of fine-needle aspiration biopsy is considered to be very small, while in core biopsies it depends on the caliber of the needle and on the organ itself. Sepsis and peritonitis are also potential complications [148]. Reports of deaths following fine-needle biopsies are very rare [35, 50, 111].

The implantation of tumor cells in the needle tract has occasionally been observed [4, 156, 158]. Apparently, this depends on the caliber of the needle and has been variously reported following perineal biopsies of prostatic carcinomas [25, 92, 97]. In fine-needle biopsies, tumor cell dissemination is an exceedingly rare complication and does not affect survival [39, 86, 160, 178]. In more than

2400 tumor patients, we have not observed a single instance of local biopsy-related metastatis. Many other authors report similar results [9, 43, 152, 158].

The suggestion of using an occluding valve in the biopsy needle to prevent tumor seeding would seem to be a rational one [151], but it appears unnecessary in view of the extreme rarity of tumor inoculation. On one occasion we accidentally punctured a hydatid cyst with a fine needle without spreading the disease or inciting an anaphylactic reaction.

Interestingly, spontaneous capillary tumor emboli may be found in the lungs and kidneys of cancer patients who show no gross evidence of metastasis. For example, cancer cell emboli have been found in the glomeruli of patients with "nonmetastasizing" carcinoma of the colon [5, 59, 144].

Apparently, the spontaneous shedding of tumor cells is observed earlier and more frequently than actual metastasis. On the one hand, the likelihood of tumor cell dissemination and the appearance of peripheral tumor emboli is influenced by tumor size, to which it is exponentially related [119, 162]. On the other hand, bone biopsies from the iliac crest may be found to contain tumor cells even in early-stage carcinoma (e.g., of the breast) before any changes appear in isotope bone scans [125].

It is clear, moreover, that fine-needle aspiration biopsies of breast or renal carcinoma have no effect on long-term survival rates [138, 167]. Also, it is safe to conclude that the inevitable injury of blood vessels by the biopsy does not contribute significantly to tumor seeding, because no increase in the rate of metastasis is observed following aspirations (e.g., of breast carcinoma) [45].

Even with melanoma, preoperative biopsy has not been shown to have a deleterious effect, assuming that definitive excision is not delayed [94].

On the basis of extensive reviews of the literature and the most recent international surveys, it may be concluded that fine-needle aspirations of the abdomen are associated with an extremely small risk of local cancer metastasis. In the review of Smith [160], for example, only three of a total of 63 108 patients were found to have metastatic deposits in the needle tract. This corresponds to a percentage of 0.005%. In the same population, the overall risk of the procedure is estimated to be 0.16%, and four deaths are reported. In another, smaller survey, local metastasis by inoculation was observed in 0.017% of the patients biopsied, with an overall risk of 0.55% – a claim that is not undisputed [97].

As a precaution, then, it has been recommended that the needle tract be excised in toto at the time of definitive surgical treatment. Certainly the very rare observation of local metastasis after biopsy does not justify abandoning this simple, rapid, inexpensive, and well-tolerated diagnostic procedure – an opinion that is shared by other authors [39, 59]. It remains to be seen whether a "safe limit" needs to be set for the maximum number of biopsies that may be performed in a given patient, and whether new needle types (thin cutting-edge needle) and techniques (rotating needle) will influence the indications for percutaneous needle biopsy.

D. Practical Aspects of Biopsy and Drainage, Indications, Risks

1 Renal Biopsy

1.1 Introduction

Certain forms of nephropathy can be accurately classified only by histopathologic means, for they are not accompanied by gross morphological changes [161] other than a reduced excretory capacity for contrast medium. These include the nephrotic syndrome (the most common renal disease affecting children), glomerulonephritis, and certain systemic diseases. In addition, ordinary diagnostic methods do not generally permit an early assessment of the progress of renal disease [41], especially in renal transplantations [132].

Even sonographic findings in the kidney are not specific for diffuse diseases, and only after initial biopsy are sonograms useful for monitoring progression of disease based on changes in renal size and cortical echo features [76].

Often the precise extent and severity of a renal disease cannot be established from hematologic and urinary findings alone, although such information is desirable and can even be essential, for example, in cases where high-dosage corticosteroid therapy is being considered. Cases of this type are an excellent indication for renal biopsy.

Successfully performed as early as the 1930s, renal biopsy was long considered a very hazardous procedure and was frequently rejected for that reason [150]. Besides the risk of infection and sepsis [142], there was concern over the danger of reflexly-induced anuria in organs with preexisting damage [6] and especially of hemorrhage – complications that still occur despite modern technical refinements [26, 116, 120, 150, 183].

The risk of renal biopsy, which was originally introduced by Iversen and Roholm as a routine study [78], has declined over the years owing to the development of percutaneous techniques that simplify the removal of tissue [77, 83]. Through the use of ultrasound guidance, which greatly aids localization of the kidneys, it is likely that the risk of biopsy will continue to decline in the future [7] and that the diagnostic yield, especially in focal diseases, will continue to improve.

1.2 Technique

Cases are selected for renal biopsy by the referring clinics in consultation with the nephrology department of our hospital. This is to ensure that the examination is limited to patients in whom the fine structure of the kidney must be known before rational therapy can be planned. This policy also extends to referring physicians and clinics abroad, who must consult with the nephrology department of our center.

The referring facility is responsible for checking laboratory values and coagulation status. One-stage prothrombin time and platelet count are routinely determined.

If hypertension exists, antihypertensive agents should be given to normalize the blood pressure before the biopsy if possible in order to reduce the risk of hemorrhage. In problem cases we conduct a repeat examination immediately prior to the biopsy.

Every percutaneous biopsy is preceded by a general ultrasound examination of the abdomen, even if this has already been done at the referring facility. Then, with the patient lying prone, both kidneys are again scanned from the posterior or posterolateral side, noting their relations to the liver and spleen. The biopsy site is dictated by the region that appears most accessible in sonograms. Generally, the needle is directed into the lower third of the kidney, giving preference to the side that is freer of overlying rib and is more easily visualized.

Once the biopsy route has been decided, the skin is antiseptically prepared and sterilely draped with a fenestrated towel, and 5–8 ml 1% lidocaine is administered for local anesthesia. No other preparations are necessary in the patient who has fasted. The biopsy transducer is held by an assistant, and the sight line of the transducer is aligned on the cortical area of the lower pole of the kidney. When the fine core needle is used, there is no need for a preliminary skin incision because the stylet-armed needle is sharp and thin enough to pass effortlessly through the skin. When a larger, blunt needle is used, such as the Tru-Cut, a preliminary skin incision is mandatory.

Under continuous sonographic guidance, the biopsy needle is advanced to a point just outside the renal capsule. The bright needle tip echo will facilitate accurate guidance. The skin offers the greatest resistance to needle insertion; the subcutaneous fat, muscle, and perirenal fat are easily penetrated. When the needle tip is within the perirenal fat but has not yet entered the capsule, the patient may safely breathe superficially under sonographic control.

The technique at this point depends on the type of needle used.

1. Tru-Cut Needle. Renal biopsy with the Tru-Cut needle (Travenol Laboratories, Illinois) is quite rapid. Also, it is reasonably certain that renal tissue will be obtained right away if the needle is used in accordance with manufacturer's recommendations. But because the tip of the Tru-Cut needle is not very echogenic and the operator must rely basically on the visible displacement of tissue layers as the needle is advanced, some degree of uncertainty exists. Moreover, we have occasionally found that the specimen contains only medullary tissue despite visual control, even when the needle is properly inserted into the cortex. This may be connected with the peculiar elasticity of the renal parenchyma.

There is no question that the larger diameter of the Tru-Cut needle carries a somewhat greater risk of hemorrhage [130]. Also, the needle cannot be advanced in apnea with the same control as finer instruments, and it may penetrate too deeply into the renal parenchyma [172].

2. Fine Core Needle. When the thin cutting-edge needle or *fine core biopsy needle* (Angiomed, D-7505 Ettlingen,) is used, the kidney itself is not punctured until the needle tip has first entered the perirenal fat. Then the biopsy is performed in several steps as previously described (see p. 84 ff).

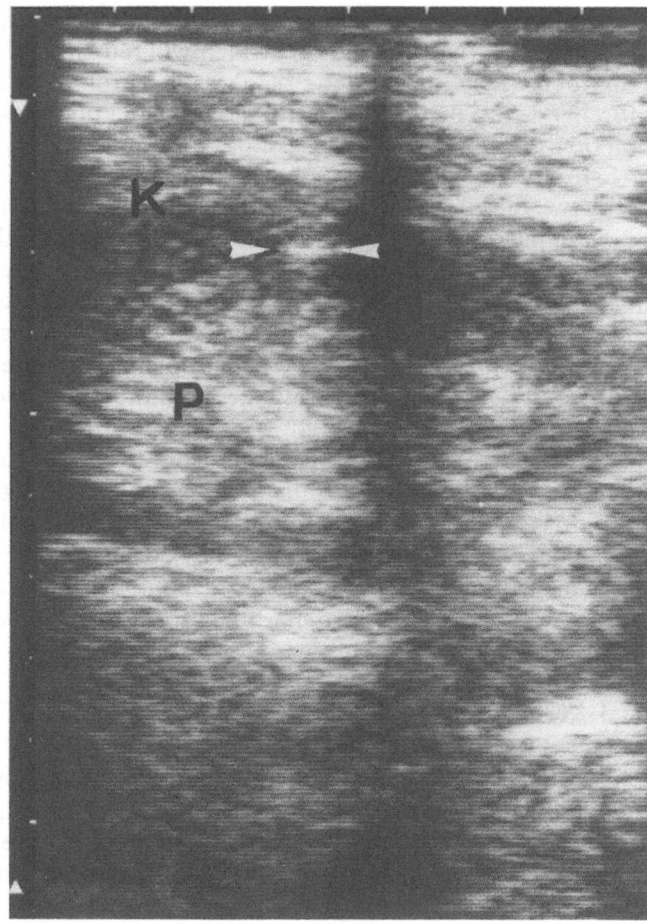

Fig. 58. Fine core biopsy of the renal cortex. The needle tip is marked with *arrows K*, cortex; *P*, renal pelvis. The biopsy needle (thin cutting-edge needle) has deviated slightly to the left of the sight line and is more visible in that position

After the stylet is removed and the syringe has been mounted and suction applied, the needle is thrust briskly into the renal cortex with a slight rotary motion while the patient suspends respiration. The good visibility of the needle tip facilitates guidance at this stage and helps to avoid inserting the needle too deeply. Because the needle is quite thin, it tends to penetrate, rather than displace, the elastic renal parenchyma. Rotation of the needle is less critical to specimen retrieval than is the brisk harpoon-like thrust of the needle into the kidney.

After perforating the renal capsule, the needle is generally moved rapidly up and down two or three times to help excise the tissue. This is the only stage of the procedure that is done in apnea; it seldom lasts more than 1s, and the needle tip remains visible at all times (Fig. 58). Once the needle has left the renal capsule, the patient may resume breathing; i.e., respiration may be resumed before the needle has left the body.

Before the needle is completely withdrawn, the suction may be released by lowering the plunger so the specimen will remain in the needle. However, passage of the material into the syringe is not a problem. Moistening the syringe beforehand with heparinized physiologic saline prevents the clotting of aspirated blood and facilitates recovery of the specimen.

In about one-third of all patients, tissue samples were obtained initially with two different needles at the same sitting (Tru-Cut needle and fine core needle). In the other patients only fine core biopsies with the thin cutting-edge needle were performed. Between two and four samples were taken at one sitting, depending on the result obtained and the length of the core.

We have not used the Vim-Silverman split needles or Menghini needles in our renal biopsies, because these instruments are more difficult to localize with ultrasound and offer no advantages, and the Vim-Silverman needle in particular is too invasive.

The biopsy core is immediately inspected with a microscope for the presence of glomeruli by a trained laboratory assistant. A special microscope should be kept ready in the examination room for just that purpose. If no glomeruli are seen, an additional sample may be taken right away. The biopsy material is placed into different fixatives, depending on the types of study proposed, and sent to the pathology department for further processing.

1.3 Postbiopsy Procedures

After the biopsy is completed, we maintain pressure on the biopsied organ (bimanually if necessary) for 5-10 min to control bleeding. In instances of sudden subcapsular hemorrhage [13], which is not entirely preventable, we have found that bleeding is satisfactorily controlled by the early and energetic use of compression.

After rechecking the status of the biopsied kidney sonographically, we turn the patient to a reclining supine position so that the pressure of the body weight is applied to the biopsy site (a sandbag is not sufficient). A hard cushion will augment this effect. Normally the patient must remain supine for at least 20 min, and preferably for 60 min.

The 24 h of bedrest formerly recommended is no longer considered necessary except in high-risk patients. After biopsies with the thin cutting-edge needle, the patient may be discharged on the same day if sonograms 2–3 h after the procedure show no abnormalities (e.g., evidence of severe hemorrhage and if there are no subjective symptoms). During the observation period, vital signs are monitored and blood pressure is checked as needed. If symptoms appear that suggest biopsy-related complications (blood loss?), the biopsied kidney is reexamined with ultrasound right away. To date only one of our patients has required postbiopsy monitoring of hemoglobin and hematocrit (see p. 111).

The complication of "delayed hemorrhage" reported in the literature should not occur with proper sonographic monitoring after biopsy. If the patient has no complaints, circulatory problems, or gross hematuria, he may be discharged home.

1.4 Results

At our hospital the ratio of renal core biopsies to fine-needle aspiration biopsies for the diagnosis of generalized parenchymal disease or tumors is approximately 1:4 at the present time. It should be noted that the indication for fine-needle aspiration of the kidney (suspected renal tumor) is recognized only by certain clinics, and that all core biopsies at our center (suspected renal inflammatory disease) are performed under ultrasound guidance.

The youngest of our patients was a 15-year-old boy, and the oldest was a 68-year-old man. Tissue samples for the three investigations – light, electron and immunofluorescent microscopy – were obtained in 89% of the biopsies. In 96% of cases a definitive diagnosis could be made on the basis of one or two microscopic techniques, however. This is consistent with the best results stated in the literature [102]. In one patient the biopsy core was inadvertently taken from the renal medulla. While the sample did not contain glomeruli, it was still possible in this instance to make a diagnosis of interstitial nephritis.

In some patients in whom repeat biopsy was contraindicated, the quantity of material obtained was insufficient for all three investigations. This did not compromise the accuracy of the diagnosis. In a few cases renal tissue was not obtained at the first attempt, and in one case the examination had to be discontinued due to lack of patient cooperation. The consistency of the organ does not significantly affect tissue removal. Failure to center the needle on the kidney, which may be abnormally mobile, makes the biopsy more difficult. Immobilization of the kidneys with a hard cushion or roll placed beneath the patient's abdomen will facilitate the procedure.

When using the thinnest cutting-edge needle with an external diameter of 0.8 mm, we repeatedly observed a peculiar effect. Rather than removing an entire tissue core, the needle selectively aspirated glomeruli, which were arranged sequentially in the specimen like a string of beads. It is still too early to decide whether the thinnest cutting-edge needle is appropriate for examinations of the renal parenchyma in all types of investigation.

We have not performed renal core biopsies under the guidance of computed tomography, because they are more costly and time-consuming [27] and require that the specimen be taken in apnea, i. e., that the needle be allowed to remain only a very short time in the organ. Also, computed-tomography-guided biopsy appears to be more hazardous because it cannot be performed under real-time guidance. In that respect it is similar to the older method of ultrasound guidance using a static scanner.

1.5 Complications and Risks

Serious complications are still reported after percutaneous renal biopsy and mainly relate to hemorrhage [16, 116, 150]. This is manifested as gross hematuria, sometimes accompanied by renal colic.

We have found transient gross hematuria to be uncommon since we began performing renal biopsies under real-time sonographic control. Presumably this is because the depth of needle penetration in the kidney can be closely monitored with ultrasound, and trauma to the calices can be avoided. Microscopic hematuria is also uncommon after ultrasound-guided biopsies.

Rarely, bleeding takes the form of a painful subcapsular hemorrhage. Bleeding of this type was difficult to detect before the development of modern imaging methods.

More dangerous are perirenal hemorrhages, the recognition of which is sometimes delayed. Children in particular are apt to show no early signs, and the danger may not be appreciated until shock and hypotension supervene [6].

Among our patients we have observed only one case of serious retroperitoneal bleeding, which occurred in a 43-year-old woman with known lupus erythematosus who had received chronic corticoid therapy (Fig. 59 a-c). Immediately after a fine core biopsy of the kidney with a 1.15-mm needle, we noted the presence of a fine, lamellar, sonolucent zone that enlarged within 10 min to an area measuring 8 cm by 2.5 cm, consistent with perirenal hemorrhage. At that time the patient reported no complaints.

Fig. 59 a-c. Incipient shrunken kidney in lupus erythematosus. a Moment of superficial insertion of the thin core needle into the renal cortex. The needle tip *(arrows)* deviates slightly from the sight line (time, 9:50; *P*, renal pelvis). b Thirteen minutes after successful biopsy, sonography shows a lamellar zone of increased sonolucency (*K*, hematoma). The kidney is displaced anteriorly. Deep respiration causes little renal movement and no movement of the hematoma. Diagnosis: child's-palm-size hematoma extending to the psoas muscle *(arrows)*. c Repeat sonogram 10 days after renal core biopsy: approximately 15-cm-long retroperitoneal hematoma of the left psoas muscle with central lamella. The normal-appearing kidney is displaced and so is not visible on this plane

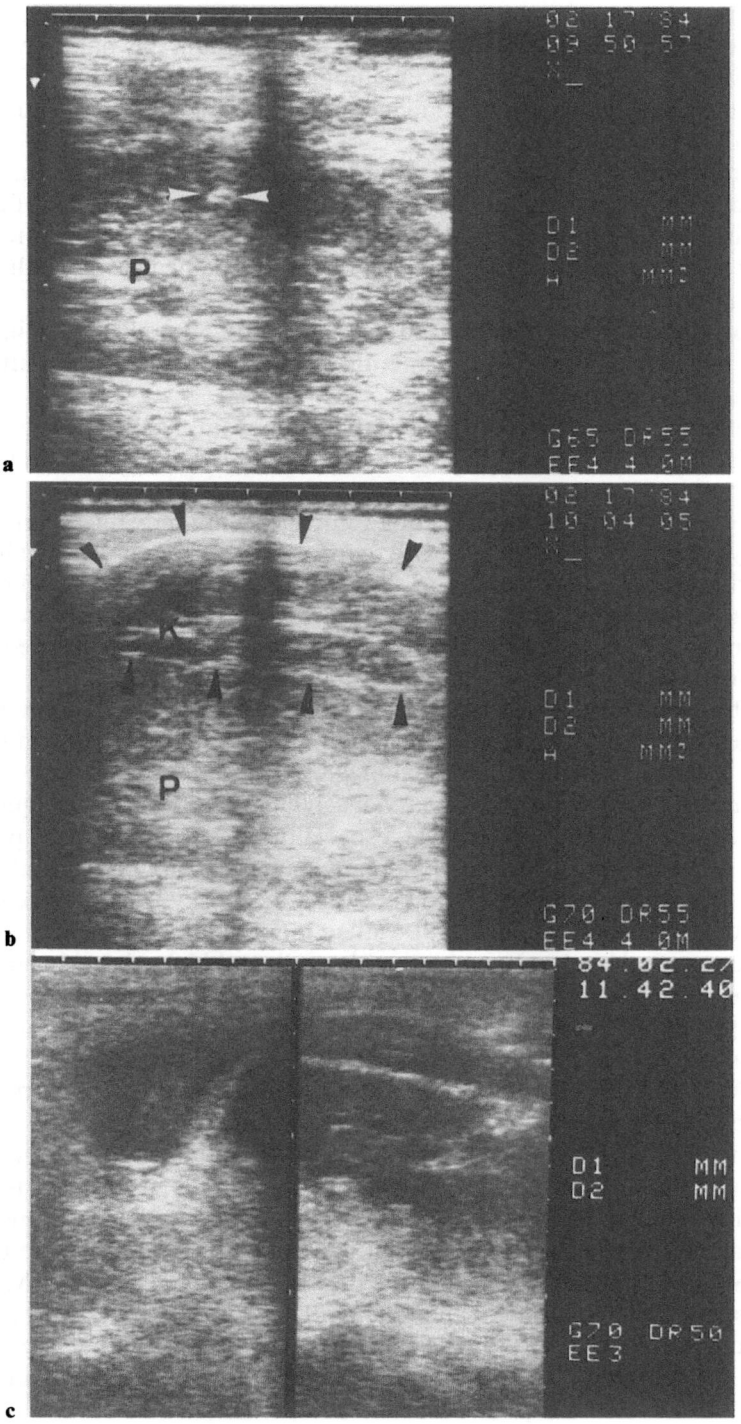

103

With prolonged bimanual compression the size of the lesion appeared to stabilize. Through a misunderstanding, compression in this patient was continued with an ineffectual sandbag. One hour later she complained of rapidly increasing pain, which at 6 h became intolerable and necessitated a morphine injection.

A repeat sonogram showed further expansion of the hematoma, which extended to the psoas muscle. Finally, it attained the size and shape of a banana. By 24 h after the biopsy clinical symptoms had largely abated, and reexamination at that time demonstrated a static but still large hematoma with indistinct margins in the left retroperitoneal area.

An ultrasound examination 10 days later (Fig. 59 c) clearly delineated the hematoma, which showed the same dimensions that it had at 6 h after biopsy and also exhibited a central lamella.

Fourteen days after biopsy the patient was completely asymptomatic and was discharged, although a residual hematoma or seroma could still be demonstrated.

Apparently, tendency to bleeding is increased not only by hypertension but also by uremia [183]. Yamauchi [179] reported a similar complication in association with nephrotic syndrome and systemic lupus erythematosus. The bleeding time and coagulation time of the patient, a 31-year-old woman, were completely normal. In our patient, retrospective study disclosed the presence of a platelet defect with a significant prolongation of bleeding time.

While emergency nephrectomies were once relatively common after renal biopsies, today they are rare, owing in part to the availability of reparative operations that can preserve renal function [95, 118].

If nephrectomy proves necessary, it can have very severe consequences that may be incompatible with survival, especially since the kidneys of patients selected for core biopsy are usually already damaged, and the contralateral kidney is often decompensated. Biopsy is also very risky in nephrotic syndrome with coexisting hypovolemia [179]. Patient inoperability is generally a contraindication to renal biopsy. In patients with a solitary kidney, it has been necessary in some cases to consider renal core biopsy following operative exposure of the organ [150], especially since the risk of the procedure is relatively low in the absence of significant uremia. The thin cutting-edge needle requires further clinical testing. But it is possible that this small-caliber needle, when correctly used, will one day expand the indications for percutaneous renal biopsy.

It is clear that complication rates are affected by the type of needle used. However, the number of patients examined to date is insufficient to permit a definitive evaluation in our series. According to data in the literature, the mortality attending of percutaneous renal biopsy ranges from 0.14% to 0.25% [88, 150]. Serious hemorrhage is described in 4%-29% of cases [116]. Most of the deaths reported to date represent individual observations that cannot be used to compute percentages. It is also clear that the complication rate is higher when an inexperienced operator performs the biopsy than when the examination is done at a center with experienced personnel.

Fistulas of the urinary tract and intrarenal arteriovenous fistulas are occasionally observed [47, 95] but will presumably become less frequent as more fine-needle biopsies are performed under ultrasound guidance. In addition, radiologic techniques are available for occluding these fistulas with a minimum of operative intervention.

In summary, then, we may say that hemorrhage remains the most significant risk of percutaneous renal biopsy. It appears that this complication cannot be entirely eliminated, even with experience and flawless technique [6, 88]. What is more, it must be acknowledged that virtually every biopsy is accompanied by small hemorrhages that are below the threshold of sonographic and computed tomographic visualization [130].

2 Liver Biopsy

2.1 Introduction

Percutaneous liver biopsy is a valuable tool in the diagnosis of certain hepatic diseases, especially the generalized types, which cannot be accurately identified by modern cross-sectional imaging methods or laboratory tests. These include certain forms of hepatitis and cirrhosis, as well as neoplasms, particularly the highly differentiated hepatoma, which is not always recognized in cytologic smears. To be effective, differentiated approaches to the treatment of hepatic insufficiency and acute hepatic failure with coma require a knowledge of the exact parameters of the quantitative functional reserve of the liver and of its regeneration [153]. It is in these cases that liver biopsy is of greatest diagnostic value.

Today liver biopsy is a routine study whose use has been greatly stimulated by the development of the Menghini needle [110]. Liver biopsy was attempted as early as the nineteenth century, but it did not gain immediate acceptance because of its hazards [99]. With improvements in technique, the risk of the procedure has diminished during the past two decades, although serious complications cannot be eliminated completely [21, 109, 155, 174]. This is due partly to the fact that smears from the liver, in contrast to smears from blood-forming organs, do not permit a morphological diagnosis of disease. Before development of the thin cutting-edge needle it was difficult to recover enough material for histologic examination. Today the mortality attending liver biopsy using standard technique is estimated to be 0.015%, with a morbidity between 0.08% [176] and 0.29% [96]. Thus, while the risk of the procedure is no longer very high, it is by no means negligible.

Given the diagnostic value of histologic specimens, it would be desirable to reduce the risk attending liver core biopsy to a level comparable to that attending fine-needle aspiration. For one thing, fine-needle aspiration can be done on an outpatient basis. For another, passage of the thin, stylet-armed needle through the skin, subcutis, peritoneum, liver capsule, and liver parenchyma traumatizes the capsule and parenchyma far less than ordinary large-bore needles, assuming that laceration of the capsule is avoided. There is no question that needle design and insertion technique affect the complication rate.

The ultrasound guidance of needle biopsy, which some clinicians consider unnecessary, removes elements of uncertainty by avoiding the inadvertent puncture of larger blood vessels and vital organs (gallbladder!) and facilitating the recognition of focal hepatic lesions whose puncture might have life-threatening consequences (necrotic tumor, hydatid cyst, hemangioma). With the danger of puncturing a major biliary duct eliminated, there is no need to fear complications such as bile peritonitis.

Computed tomography is also used to guide liver biopsies but is more costly and time-consuming and, we feel, more hazardous than sonographic guidance.

In the search for an instrument that would yield sufficient material for histologic evaluation while minimizing trauma to the capsule, we developed a small-caliber cutting-edge needle which provides a very thin but elongated core of tissue. With this needle it is possible to retrieve histologic specimens from the liver, kidneys, and other internal organs, and the failure rate of the instrument is practically nil. Figure 52 a shows three core specimens taken from the liver. The specimen on the right was obtained with the thin cutting-edge needle (external diameter 0.8 mm). It is more than 15 mm long. On the left is the shorter, thicker core obtained with a Tru-Cut needle 2.1 mm in diameter. Both specimens are adequate for histologic diagnosis. So far we have observed no significant postbiopsy hemorrhage in ultrasound or computed tomography scans, although a few patients have reported brief episodes of pain. Operative intervention has not been required, and none of the patients have required later hospitalization.

Because the thin cutting-edge needle is still new, we have been able to use it in only a limited number of patients (about 350). Thus, experience acquired to date needs to be confirmed in a larger patient population. Nevertheless, we are convinced that liver core biopsies with the thin needle can almost always be done on an outpatient basis when followed by 30-90 min observation (cf. [44, 134]) and a final ultrasound examination.

The minimum needle diameter of 1.5-2 mm advocated by some clinicians [99, 176] is certainly too great in view of the most recent techniques. The advantages of a smaller needle are obvious: reduced risk and increased patient acceptance.

It should be added that biopsies of blood-rich organs like the liver necessarily carry a certain risk that warrants caution. The reputed "safety" of liver biopsy should not tempt the physician to underestimate its risks. This especially applies to seriously ill patients who are not good candidates for surgery.

2.2 Technique

First the liver is scanned for the presence of focal abnormalities. If none are found, but a generalized parenchymal change is noted, a biopsy site is selected that is readily accessible and shows the least respiratory movement. The preferred site for liver biopsy is the left lobe, because it reduces the risk of capsular injury even in uncooperative patients, and the needle can be maneuvered somewhat more freely than between the ribs. In addition, that is the only area that allows compression of the biopsy site.

If the left lobe is very small, or if the liver is located high in the thorax, the only remaining option is the intercostal route, but this presents no significant problems when sonographic guidance is used.

It should be noted that the right intercostal approach is basically more hazardous than a left-lobe biopsy, and that some two-thirds of fatal hemorrhages reported in the literature have been associated with intercostal biopsies [99]. However, these incidents occurred before the advent of diagnostic ultrasound, and thus at a time when physicians were unfamiliar with ultrasound-guided biopsy, used relatively large-gauge needles, and apparently gave little attention to coagulation times.

With the transducer accurately positioned over the organ, the sight line is directed past the major blood vessels and bile ducts so that these structures will be missed when the needle is inserted.

Two different techniques are available for obtaining the biopsy:

1. The thin cutting-edge needle with indwelling stylet is inserted through the skin and subcutaneous tissue but is stopped before piercing the peritoneum. At this point the stylet is removed, the syringe is mounted, and a vacuum (5 ml) is produced.
   The patient suspends respiration and, under sonographic vision, the needle is quickly thrust through the peritoneum and liver capsule into the hepatic tissue and is immediately withdrawn from the body. The actual excision of tissue takes about 1 s.
2. The thin cutting-edge needle with indwelling stylet is inserted through the skin, subcutaneous fat, peritoneum, and liver capsule into the parenchyma. Then the stylet is removed, the syringe is mounted, and the specimen is taken as described above.

The thin cutting-edge needle is fairly elastic, depending on its exact caliber, so it is able to follow an involuntary movement of the liver, such as that caused by a deep, involuntary inspiration, to a certain degree if it has been inserted deeply enough into the tissue (at least 2–3 cm). A laceration of the capsule caused by a needle tip inserted to a depth of only a few millimeters can be extremely dangerous. Consequently, the needle should be advanced into the liver rapidly and to a depth of 2–3 cm.

Any unexpected movement of the organ, incidentally, can be seen at once on the ultrasound monitor, enabling the operator to withdraw the needle at once if necessary. The depth of insertion is 2–5 cm, or somewhat more with focal lesions. This superficial insertion will generally yield enough material for histologic study. Cores obtained by this method are up to 3 cm in length and permit a full histologic evaluation, especially since there is no problem with crushing of the specimen, such as that occurs with other biopsy needles.

If the tissue is densely fibrotic, as in certain forms of cirrhosis, it is best to use a cutting-edge needle with an external diameter of 0.95 mm or 1.2 mm. However, the attempt to take the biopsy with the smallest-caliber needle is worthwhile, as it will usually provide an adequate specimen while creating a minimal needle track.

2.3 Results

In all cases the thin cutting-edge needle retrieved representative tissue from the liver. This is accomplished very easily with the largest-caliber needle (external diameter 1.15 mm) and, with some practice, with the smallest-caliber needle as well (external diameter 0.78 mm).

Most core biopsies were done in patients with suspected generalized hepatic parenchymal disease (fatty liver, alcoholic cirrhosis, hemosiderosis, etc.). In a few cases we biopsied suspicious intrahepatic focal lesions where prior fine-needle aspiration had failed to identify the mass, as in hepatoma or in focal steatosis, which has a tumor-like sonographic appearance.

In seven patients we had to perform two core biopsies during the initial trial period, apparently because the specimen was retained in the needle tract during the first biopsy. Since then we have adopted the practice of maintaining suction even while the needle is removed from the body. Often this draws the biopsy core into the syringe, but it is easily flushed out with physiologic saline. This method saves time: the biopsy can be taken literally in a matter of seconds.

In the first patients biopsied, the fine core biopsy was followed by a second fine core biopsy at the same location or by a biopsy with the Tru-Cut needle. This gave us a chance to compare the two needles with regard to tissue yield.

Recently we changed from the largest-caliber cutting-edge needle to the thinnest caliber for routine liver biopsies. Even with the thinnest needle a histologic diagnosis can almost always be established without difficulty once the pathologist becomes accustomed to working with the smaller quantity of material.

In the cirrhotic liver preference is given to the next larger needle size (0.95 mm), because a reasonably complete examination of the portal fields is necessary for accurate interpretation. Clockwise rotation of the needle as it enters the hepatic tissue is less important to retrieving a good sample than a rapid thrust of the needle to a depth of 2–3 cm from the capsular margin, assuming an ordinary tissue consistency.

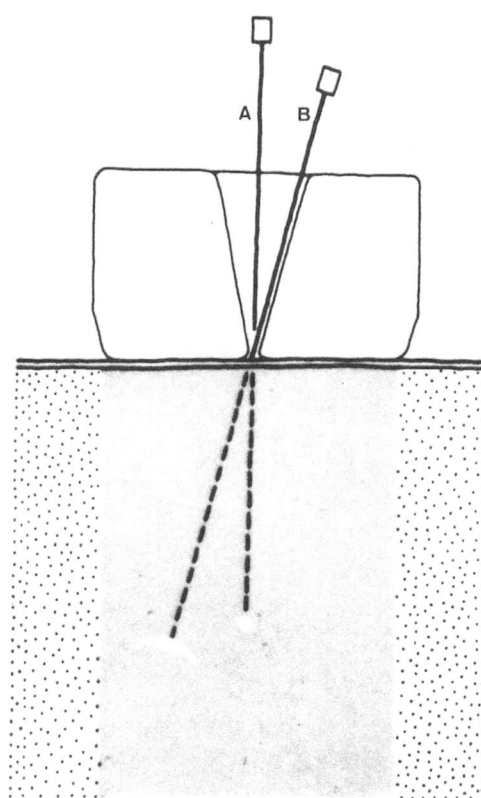

Fig. 60. Recommended angles of needle insertion through the apertured transducer. *A*, fine-needle aspiration, vertical insertion; *B*, core biopsy, e.g., with thin cutting-edge needle, slightly oblique insertion

Care is taken to introduce the needle at a slight angle to the sight line of the transducer. In this way even a larger-gauge needle will remain clearly visible throughout the procedure. In diffuse parenchymal diseases, this slight deviation from the sight line will not affect diagnostic yield (Figs. 60 and 61).

To date we have experienced no complications in fine core biopsies of the liver. Nevertheless, we are aware that the potential for complications in liver biopsies always exists (see Sect. 2.4). Further studies are necessary in larger patient groups before a final evaluation of the needle can be made.

2.4 Complications and Risks

Like the success rate in retrieving useful histologic samples, the complication rate of liver core biopsies is accurately known and has been investigated in various studies [58, 108, 182]. Pain, hemorrhage, and hypotension are the complications most frequently described [134]. As one would expect, the experience of the operator has a greater bearing on the risk of complications than does needle

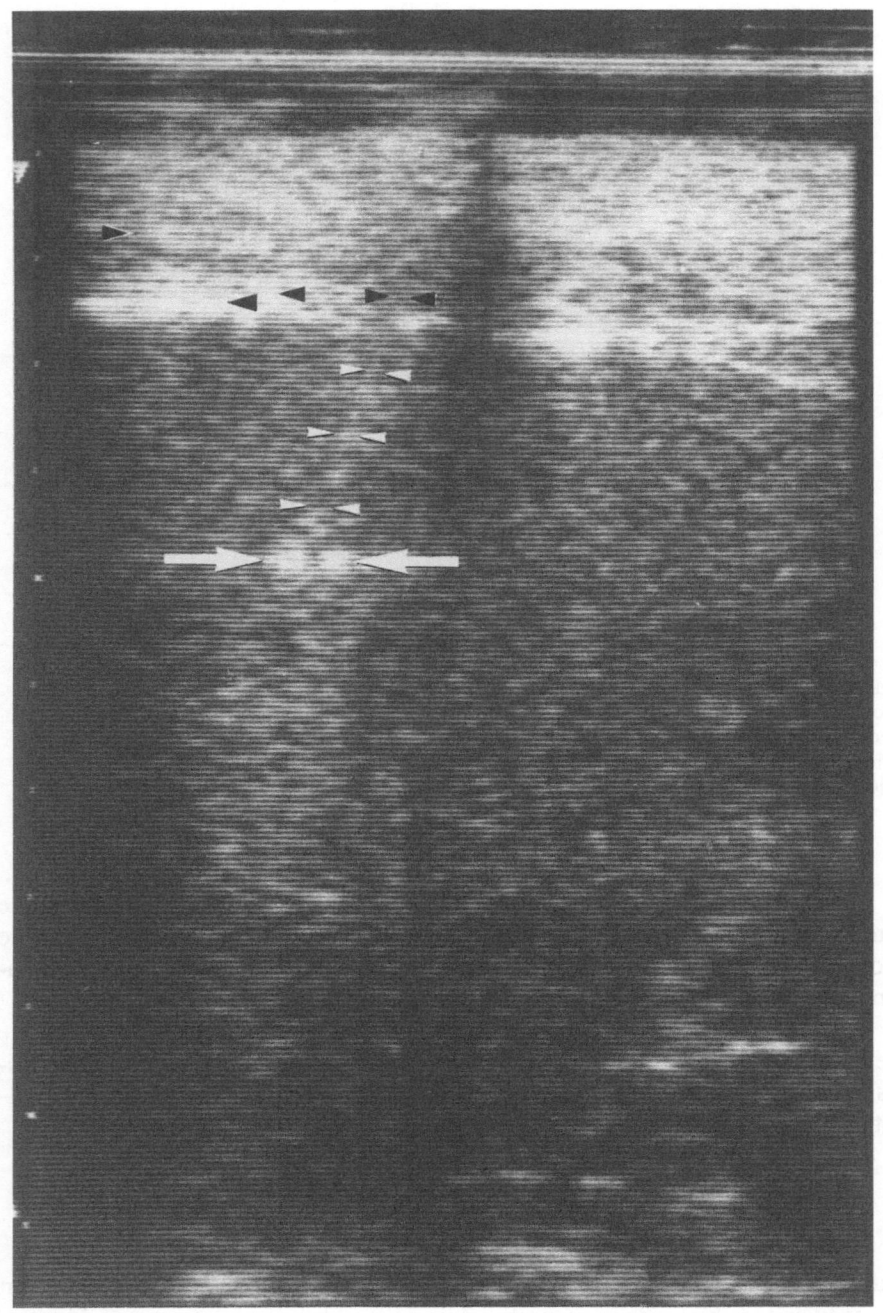

Fig. 61. Ultrasound-guided core biopsy of the liver. The thin cutting-edge needle has been intro-duced at a slight angle to the sight line for better visualization in the tissue. The needle tip is marked with *large arrows.* The usual, adequate depth of needle insertion into the liver *(centimeter scale at left edge of picture)* is 2–3 cm *(small arrows:* needle shaft)

selection, although animal experiments in the open abdomen show a marked correlation between tendency to bleeding and the type of needle used [130]. But if the external diameter of the needle is a factor in the risk of hemorrhage [22], one must necessarily give preference to an instrument with the smallest possible diameter that still allows a meaningful histologic assessment.

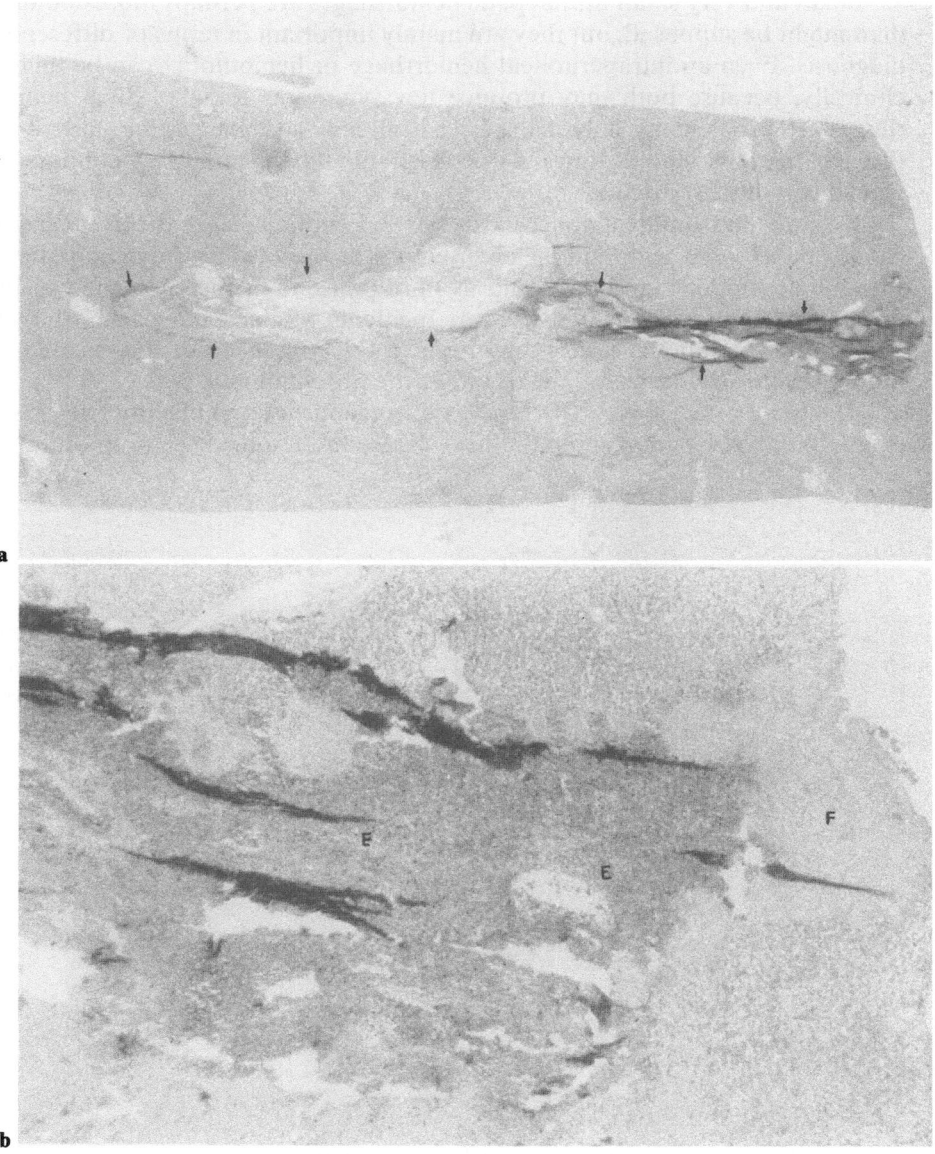

Fig. 62a,b. Liver biopsy. **a** Needle tract *(arrows)* after biopsy with a Tru-Cut needle. **b** End of needle tract at the surface of the liver. Erythrocytes *(E)* and fibrin masses *(F)* completely fill the tract

Hemorrhage. Extravasated blood has a tendency to spread within the liver and may be clinically silent. A fall of hematocrit and changes in serum hepatic enzyme levels are indicative of such a complication [22]. Intrahepatic hemorrhages can be detected by scintigraphy because they inhibit radionuclide uptake by the parenchyma, but today this method has been superseded by sonography and computed tomography.

Small and very small intrahepatic hemorrhages are perhaps more common than might be supposed, but they are mainly important in terms of differential diagnosis. Even an intraperitoneal hemorrhage or hemothorax can be missed clinically, because both may produce few symptoms initially. Such hemorrhages are problematic only if the liver is already so damaged by underlying disease that it is tending toward necrosis, and a hematoma can continue to spread with little restriction.

Despite ultrasound guidance of the biopsy needle, a tear of the liver capsule cannot be avoided with complete certainty, for there will always be patients who inhale suddenly and involuntarily in response to the needle pain, causing an associated movement of the liver. Incidents of this kind can be largely avoided by the rational use of anesthesia, a brisk insertion of the needle (see Sect. 2.2), and withdrawal of the needle at the proper time.

The biopsy needle leaves behind a conspicuous tract in healthy liver tissue (Fig. 62 a,b), yet bleeding from the liver ceases more quickly than in other or-

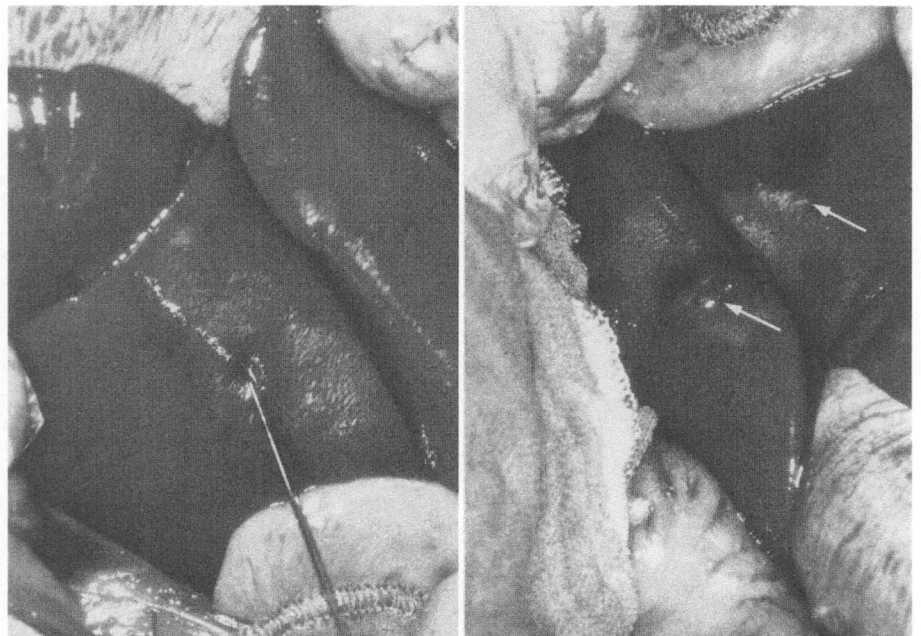

a   b

Fig. 63 a,b. Biopsy of both lobes of the liver. **a** Insertion of the thin cutting-edge needle into the left lobe. **b** Twenty seconds after second core biopsy. Bleeding from the needle tracts is slight *(arrows)* and ceases without compression

gans such as the kidney, apparently because hepatic blood coagulates very rapidly. This is known to surgeons and can be demonstrated in laboratory animals (see Fig. 63 a,b).

Other complications consist of arteriovenous fistulas or septic febrile episodes. Apparently, fistulas between the hepatic arteries and portal vein system are not uncommon according to computed tomographic investigations, but they have little if any clinical significance. Also, radiologic methods are available for closing these fistulas without operative intervention.

Liver biopsy by the transjugular route is an involved procedure whose potential late complications contraindicate its use except in cases where it is performed concurrently with cholangiography.

In about one-third of all patients with a hepatic disease that requires a histologic diagnosis, factors are present which contraindicate percutaneous liver biopsy. In these cases transvenous liver biopsy provides an acceptable alternative.

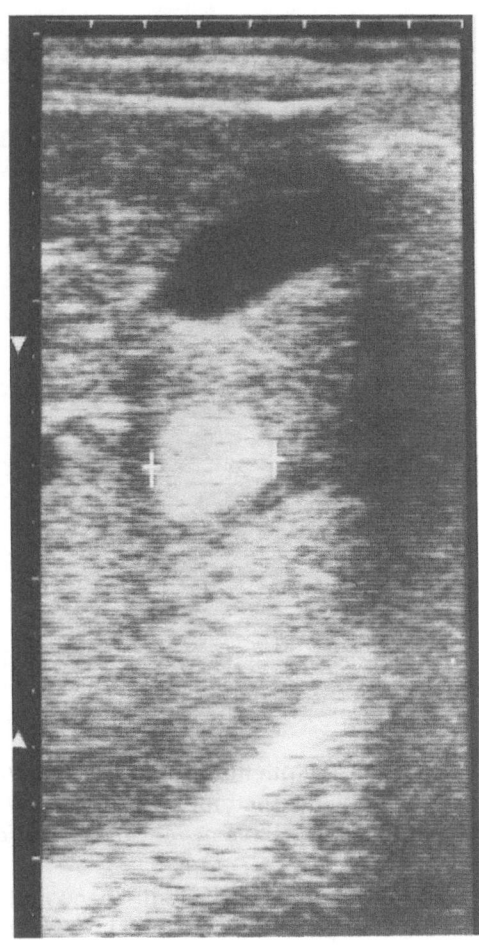

Fig. 64. Capillary hemangioma, presenting as a bright, hyperechoic mass through the "window" of the gallbladder

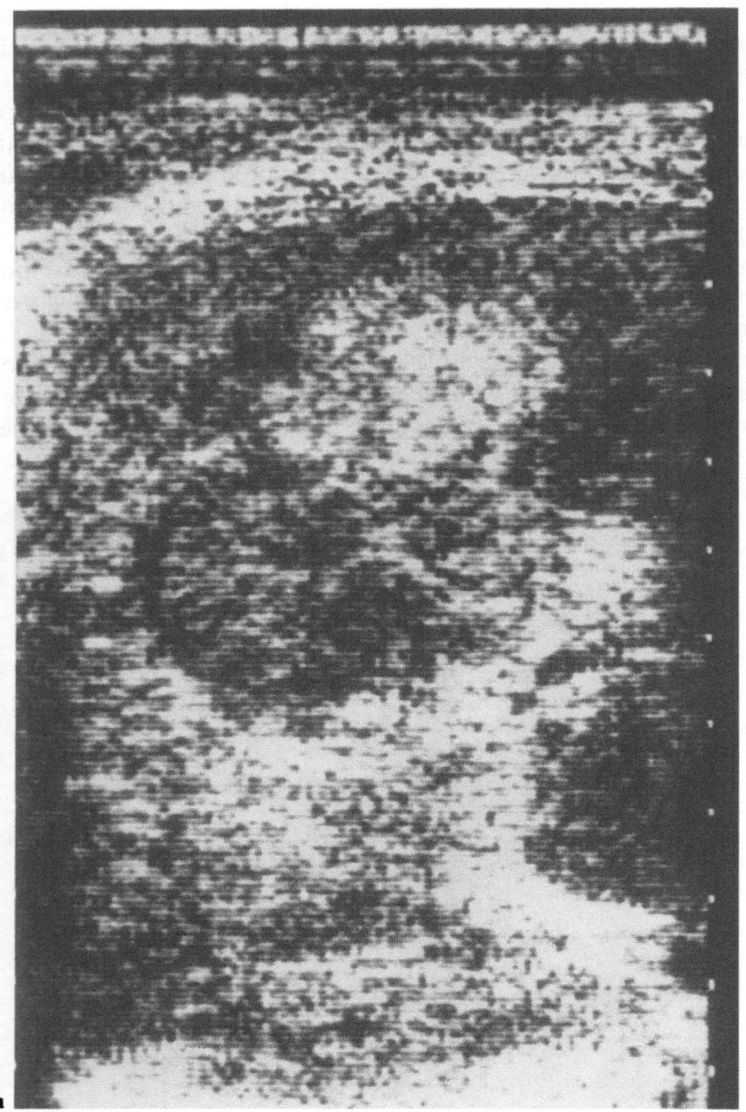

a

Fig. 65 a-c. Large, cavernous hemangiomas of the liver. **a** Sonographic differential diagnosis: hematoma. **b** Computed tomographic scan in the same patient, early injection phase. **c** Late phase with centripetal flow of contrast material

Pleuritis, pneumothorax, and subcutaneous emphysema can reportedly be avoided when the biopsy is guided by cross-sectional imaging. However, these complications have never posed a serious threat to patients.

Hypotension. It is difficult to account for the hypotension that sometimes occurs after percutaneous liver biopsy. Because it is accompanied by bradycardia,

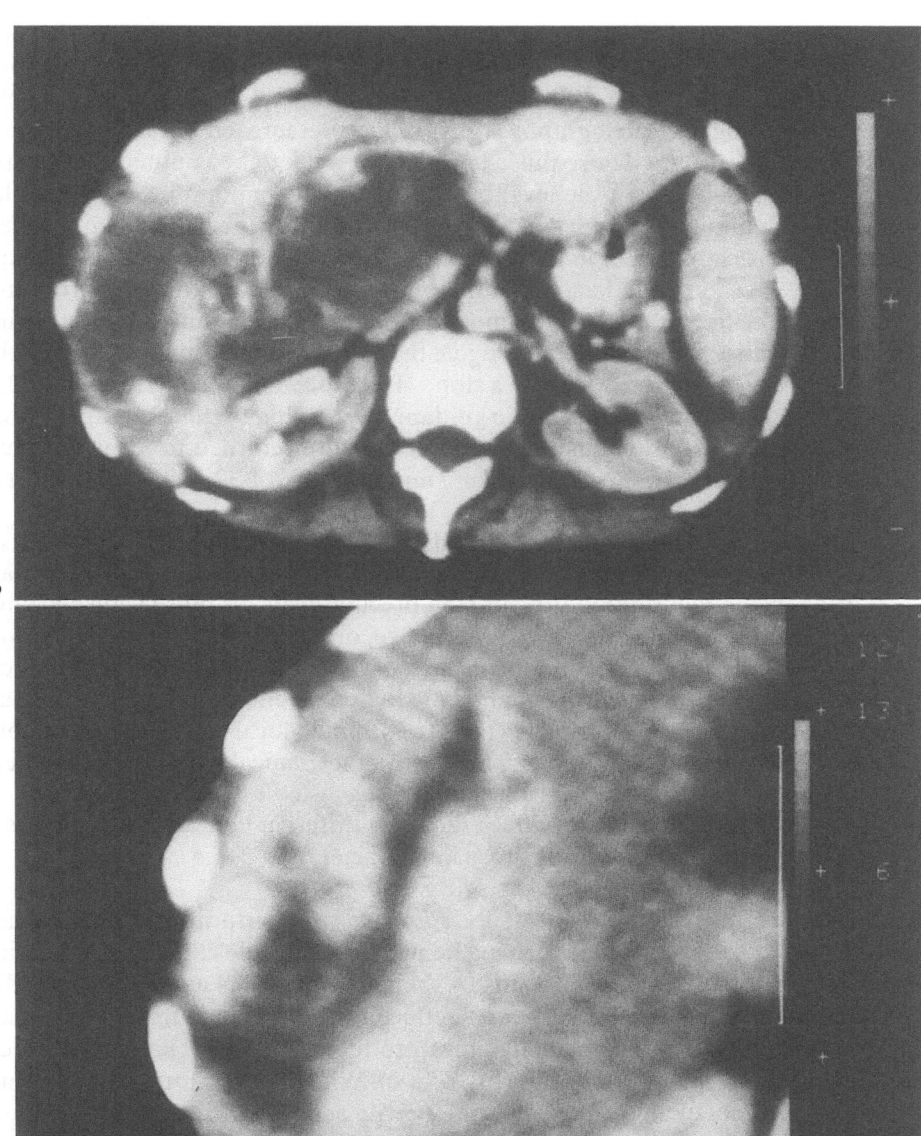

b

c

it cannot be related to blood loss, and apparently it is referrable to vagus nerve stimulation [8, 24, 36]. Usually the hypotension regresses without treatment, although fatal outcomes have been described in the literature [13, 164, 182].

A hypotensive reaction accompanied by an accelerated pulse must have a different etiologic mechanism, such as the release of endotoxins in the presence of an occult infection [139].

115

Among the more than 3000 patients biopsied at our center, and among 600 liver biopsies performed mostly with aspiration needles but also with various core needles, we have observed one severe hypotensive crisis in a 62-year-old man undergoing cholangiography whose blood pressure temporarily fell below measurable levels and whose pulse became too weak to be counted. Following a fine-needle puncture at the level of the proximal common bile duct with the injection of contrast medium and a slight extravasation, the patient experienced sudden, excruciating pain in that region and lost consciousness for almost half a minute. A scan of the heart with the biopsy transducer showed a profound slowing of the heart rate. The common bile duct had been punctured for the injection of contrast material to investigate the cause of an intermittent biliary obstruction, which later proved to be a stone. The procedure was performed under sonographic and then fluoroscopic guidance according to the technique previously described [129]. The patient's blood pressure returned to normal within 20 min. The bradycardia persisted for 7 min at a rate of 32/min, afterward increasing to 56/min.

Another patient was undergoing a fine-needle aspiration biopsy of a fist-sized malignant liver tumor. When the needle accidentally punctured the hepatic portal, the patient's blood pressure fell precipitously, his pulse vanished, and he temporarily lost consciousness. We believe, on the basis of our own observations, that these reactions were the product of a typical vagus nerve stimulation corresponding to the "neurogenic hepatic hypotension" described by Sullivan and Watson [164]. The most likely cause was a small, local extravasation of contrast material (mixed with bile?) or possibly a mechanical irritation by the needle tip, rather than the "liver displacement" suggested by some authors.

A local bile peritonitis produces radically different clinical symptoms, is a later occurrence, and is not transitory in character.

Puncture of Hemangioma. Repeatedly, surgeons who perform liver biopsies are warned of the danger of puncturing a hemangioma. While capillary hemangiomas are distinguished in sonograms by their sharp borders and their markedly dense, homogeneous echo structure, reflecting the architecture of the lesion (Fig. 64), larger cavernous hemangiomas produce a hypoechoic pattern which mimics that of a malignant tumor (Fig. 65 a-c). With a satisfactory platelet count and normal coagulation times, the fine-needle aspiration of a hemangioma is not considered particularly dangerous, and we personally have encountered no problems in more than 50 aspirations of hepatic hemangiomas. This applies with equal validity to biopsies with the thin cutting-edge needle. Reports of fatal outcomes after hemangioma biopsies are exceptional [50].

The safest method of biopsying lesions that extend to the surface of the organ or into the liver capsule is to introduce the needle somewhat obliquely and from the side, so that the needle traverses a zone of normal hepatic tissue before entering the lesion (Fig. 66). In this way the elastic intervening tissue will seal the needle tract after the biopsy and prevent hemorrhage. This technique also helps to avoid tearing of the capsule by a thin needle at the point of least resi-

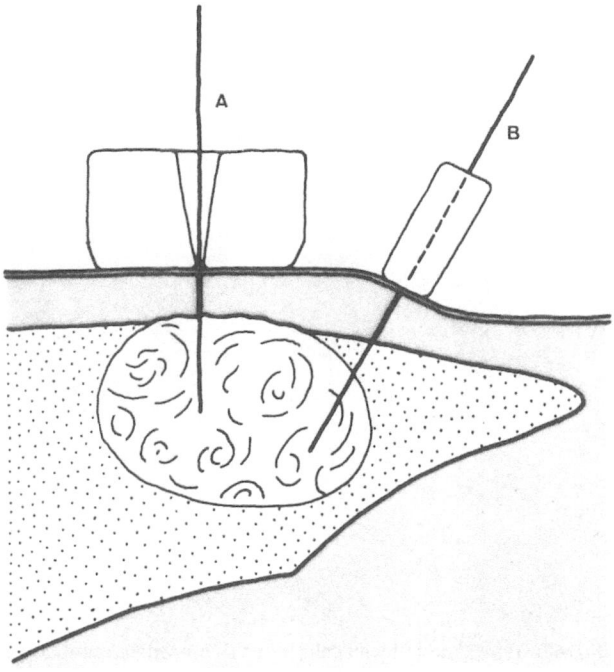

Fig. 66. With a space-occupying lesion extending to the surface of the liver, an "oblique" biopsy through a mantle of normal tissue *(B)* is advised. Direct biopsy *(A)* carries a greater risk of capsule laceration and hemorrhage

stance caused by a sharp, involuntary inspiration as the needle enters the organ.

Rarely, a capillary hemangioma will lose its normal echogenic structure after biopsy and will present as a dark, hypoechoic zone. This is caused by a circumscribed hemorrhage within the hemangioma itself and is a transient phenomenon, seldom lasting more than an hour.

To obtain site-specific material from a hemangioma, the needle must be inserted into the lesion with a quick thrust under low suction. In this way endothelial cells can be obtained with minimum aspiration of blood (Fig. 67). There are authors who consider the diagnosis of hemangioma to be established when only blood is aspirated from a lesion that has the sonographic features of a hemangioma. However, problems of differentiation may arise in connection with certain types of metastatic tumor, especially carcinomas of the intestinal tract, which appear highly echogenic.

Cavernous hemangiomas can also be detected with angiography and computed tomography. Computed tomographic scans of these lesions show a characteristic centripetal uptake of contrast material. However, the costs of both methods are considerable, and radiation exposure is unavoidable (Fig. 65 b,c).

Of course, we avoid the use of larger-gauge needles like the Tru-Cut when performing core biopsies of hemangiomas, and we caution against their use be-

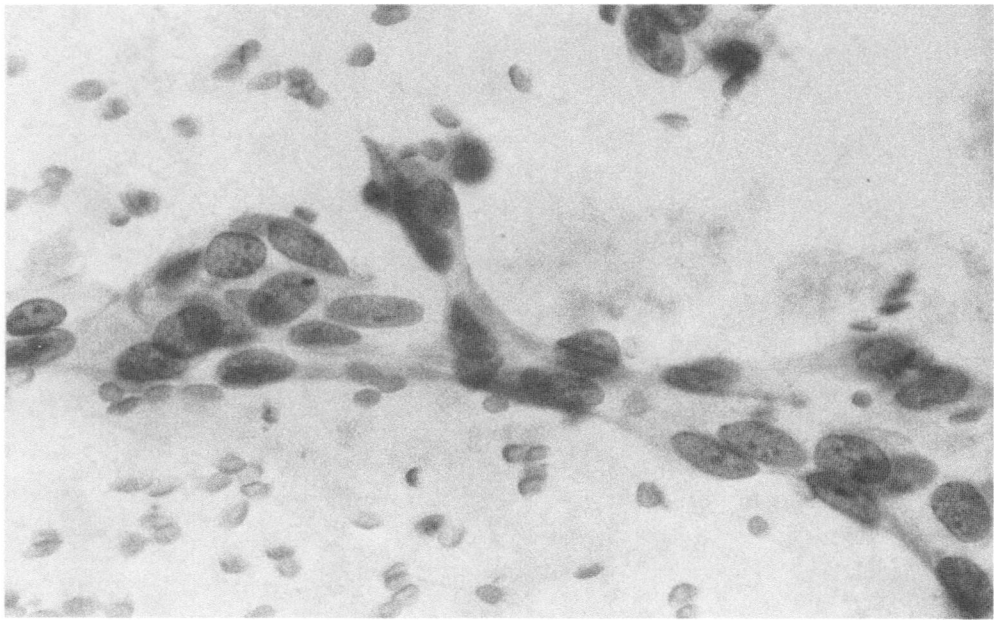

Fig. 67. Typical endothelial cells in the fine-needle aspirate from a hemangioma. × 600

cause of the unacceptably high risk. Our standard procedure for circumscribed hepatic lesions is the fine-needle aspiration biopsy or possibly a fine core biopsy, which is supplemented if necessary by a more extensive core biopsy at a second sitting (e.g., in cases where computed tomographic findings are unclear). This has rarely been necessary, however.

2.5 Contraindications

The contraindications to liver biopsy derive in part from the complications described earlier. They will be reviewed briefly below. Biopsies with the fine core needle no longer differ significantly from aspiration biopsies, which use only a slightly smaller needle caliber.

Contraindications to liver core biopsy are:
1. Increased tendency to bleeding
2. Cardiac decompensation with hepatic congestion
3. Obstructive jaundice (risk of peritonitis!)
4. Inflammations of biliary passages or of the liver itself (abscess)
5. (In intercostal biopsy) diseases of the right lower lobe of the lung and pulmonary emphysema.

When ultrasound guidance is used, exceptions may be made in cases 3–5 above.

The minumum blood coagulation standards ordinarily required in biopsy candidates (one-stage prothrombin 50%, platelet count 80000–100000/mm^2) may be relaxed somewhat if the indication for a pathologic diagnosis appears urgent. However, the concomitant presence of right heart failure with hepatic congestion is an absolute contraindication to liver core biopsy.

The perforation of a superficial, dilated bile duct can be avoided with the help of continuous ultrasound guidance. The insertion of a thin needle into the biliary tract through a mantle of intact parenchyma prevents bile leakage owing to spontaneous and immediate closure of the needle tract.

We have not yet encountered massive bile peritonitis of the type described in the literature [99]. It is a grave complication that is fatal in the overwhelming majority of cases. The risk of this complication should be very small when a thin needle is used and care is taken to avoid the accidental puncture of large bile ducts or the gallbladder.

Hepatic abscess is no longer an absolute contraindication to needle biopsy. True peritonitis is avoidable as long as the abscess is not punctured at its junction with the surface of the liver. The needle should traverse at least a 1-cm mantle of normal liver tissue before entering the abscess, employing a longer or more oblique biopsy route as needed (Fig. 66).

Even pulmonary emphysema is only a relative contraindication, since perforation of the lung is easily avoided under sonographic vision, and air should not enter the pleural space if the procedure is correctly planned.

2.6 Echinococcosis

All surgical textbooks caution categorically against the percutaneous puncture of a hydatid cyst, even with a fine-gauge needle, because of the danger of anaphylactic shock and the possibility of disseminating the disease. This is basically a good rule to follow [113], although occasionally scolices and hooklets are discovered fortuitously in hepatic aspirates [49, 80], as every performer of fine-needle biopsies is aware. Remarkably, the majority of these aspirations go better than expected, although instances of unusual clinical behavior after the biopsies have been interpreted as evidence of anaphylactoid reaction.

If sonograms disclose a lesion of the type shown in Fig. 68, caution is advised. The cystic, septate mass is typical of the vesicle with daughter cysts produced by *Echinococcus granulosis*. It was discovered as an "incidental finding" in a 43-year-old Spanish woman with unexplained abdominal complaints (Fig. 68).

Differences in the intensity of reactions to surgical procedures or punctures of hydatid cysts probably relate to differences in the release of antigen, which in turn depends on the integrity of the parasite wall or previous episodes of trauma [20].

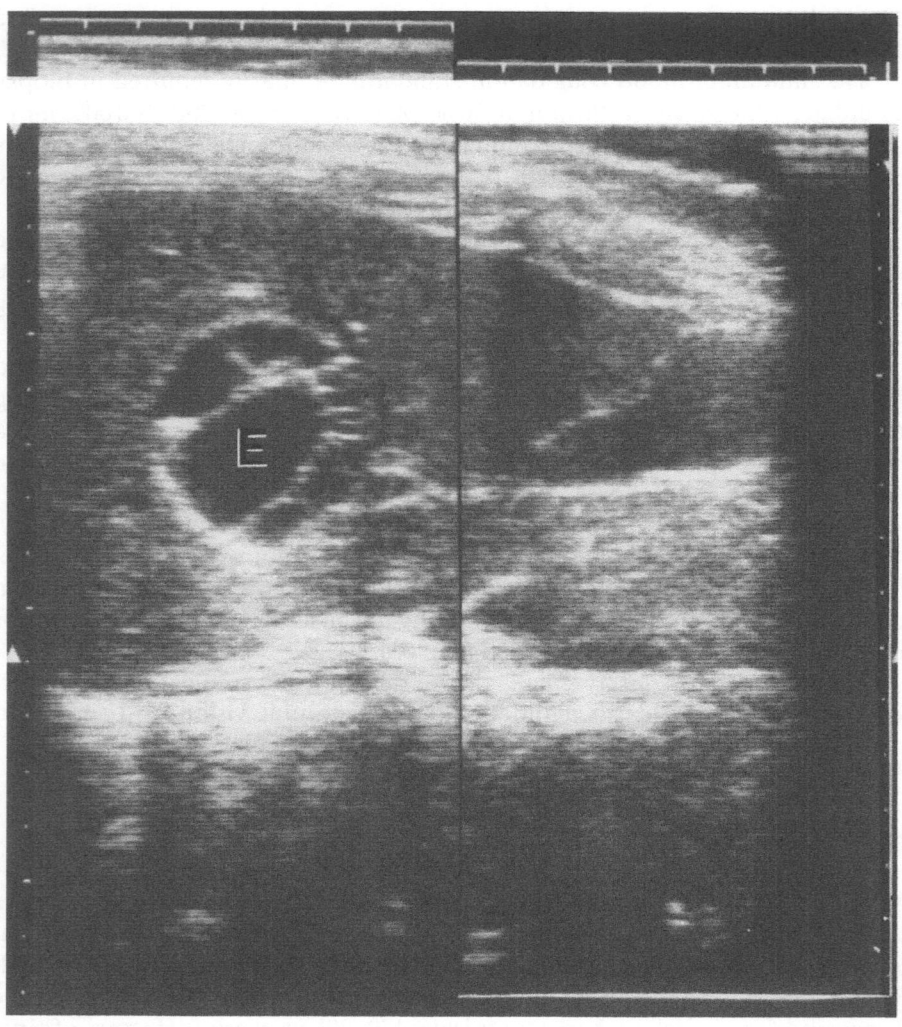

Fig. 68. *Echinococcus granulosus (cysticus).* Incidental finding in a 43-year-old Spanish woman

There have been numerous reports from Turkey on percutaneous fine-needle aspirations of hydatid cysts [154]. The lesions were either punctured inadvertently because they could not be distinguished from banal cysts, or they were aspirated intentionally without provoking serious symptoms, since "extravasation does not occur with proper aspirating technique." On the basis of these experiences, it has even been suggested that in certain cases, scolicidal agents should be injected directly into the hydatid cyst under sonographic control.

Serious sequelae after the surgical treatment of hepatic echinococcosis are well known [2], but apparently only the spontaneous rupture of the host capsule

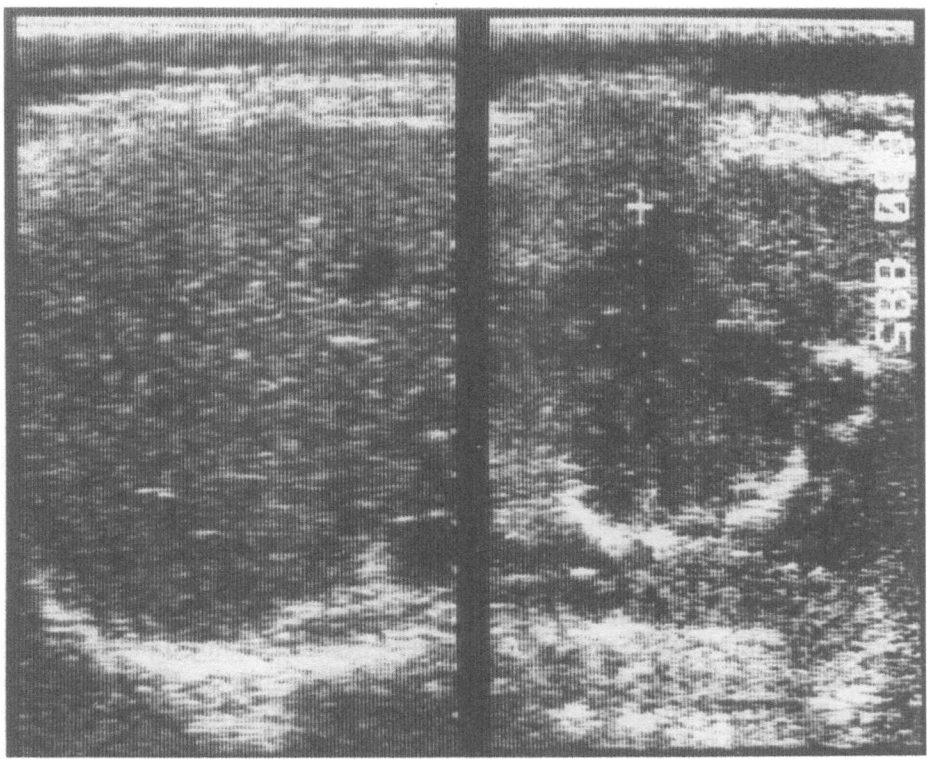

Fig. 69. *Echinococcus multilocularis (alveolaris).* The echogenic mass *(crosses)* mimics the appearance of a neoplasm

is particularly dangerous. Moreover, spillage of the cyst contents does not invariably elicit a life-threatening anaphylactic reaction [60], even with rupture into the biliary tract [146].

The lesions of *Echinococcus multilocularis* mimic a hepatic tumor. A typical pattern is seen in Fig. 69. In the later stage these masses show a cyst-like degeneration with a wide, echogenic margin, but in the early stage they are indistinguishable from metastases. They behave similarly to malignant neoplasms and tend to expand past organ boundaries. On initial evaluation, even computed tomography and sonography may fail to establish a diagnosis, especially if typical calcifications are absent. Usually, the initial impression is of a primary hepatic tumor [131]. Even intraoperative diagnosis can be difficult [84]. Fine-needle aspiration, performed with the same precautions as those observed for a suspected hemangioma, is reasonably safe, and anaphylactic reactions should not be a problem. One such successful puncture is described in the literature [159]. Seeding of echinococcosis into the needle tract remains a potential danger, however.

If the parasite has already infiltrated the diaphragm, retroperitoneum, or inferior vena cava, with concomitant thrombosis of that vessel, fine-needle aspiration is unnecessary since the identity of the disease is known.

The benefit of a liver biopsy (and of punctures in general) must always be weighed against the risk of complications. But if a microscopic examination of biopsy material is considered to be of vital importance to the patient, a biopsy is not only justified but imperative.

3 Percutaneous Nephrostomy

3.1 Introduction

Thirty years ago the technique of percutaneous nephrostomy was developed from percutaneous antegrade pyelography as a means of identifying the cause of a urinary tract obstruction and providing temporary or permanent decompression of the affected kidney [55, 128, 169, 173]. Generally, the procedure was done strictly as an emergency measure to prevent impending uremia and irreversible renal damage. Today the indications for percutaneous nephrostomy are considerably broader, owing to improvements in technique. For example, in patients with a ureteropelvic stenosis, percutaneous nephrostomy may be used in conjunction with the Whitacker test to assess the recovery potential of the renal parenchyma before pyeloplasty is attempted [61].

With the development of computed tomography and sonography and the availability of improved catheter materials, percutaneous nephrostomy has become a routine measure that is well tolerated by patients and is being utilized with increasing frequency [65, 105, 128, 177]. Complications have become progressively less frequent, although they have not been entirely eliminated.

Indications

The indications for percutaneous pyelostomy are numerous and may be classified as diagnostic or therapeutic.

Main Indications for Percutaneous Pyelonephrostomy

1. Diagnostic
   Antegrade pyelography
   Brush biopsy of ureteropelvic and caliceal lesions
   Assessment of potential for functional recovery of obstructed kidney
   (Whitacker test)
   Percutaneous nephroscopy.

122

2. Therapeutic
   Decompression of vesical or supravesical urinary tract obstruction
   Percutaneous urinary diversion in the presence of urinary fistula (e.g., of the ureter)
   Placement of stent
   Drainage of pyonephrosis
   Extraction of renal and ureteral stones
   Lithotripsy
   Ureteral embolization.

Percutaneous nephrostomy is the primary measure for various endourologic manipulations and exists in various modifications. The removal of renal and ureteral calculi represents a new application that will almost certainly gain in importance with passage of time. In view of its safety and relative simplicity, the insertion of a drainage catheter into the renal pelvis under sonographic guidance is gaining increasing clinical acceptance [124, 128, 143].

Most nephrostomies in the past were performed under fluoroscopic control [106, 141]. Drawing on existing systems, we have developed new nephrostomy sets [65, 128] that can be directed into the renal pelvis under either sonographic or radiologic control and have a variety of other applications (e.g., drainage of abscesses or biliary tract). With these new sets the renal pelvis can be catheterized quickly and at very little risk.

A major improvement relates to the use of a catheter material that can be left indwelling for a prolonged period without aging or encrustation. A drainage catheter produced from this material has been commercially available for about 3 years (Angiomed, D-7505 Ettlingen) and has proved its efficacy for long-term diversion of the kidney.

3.2 Technique

There are two basic techniques of ultrasound-guided nephrostomy, one involving *indirect insertion* of the nephrostomy tube over a guide wire as in the Seldinger technique, and the other involving *direct insertion* of the tube over a stabilizing needle. The choice of technique will depend on individual factors, especially the degree of dilatation of the renal collecting system and the accessibility of the kidney (overlying ribs, obesity, etc.). Indirect nephrostomy is the method of choice when there is minimum dilatation of the pyelocaliceal system. It is less hazardous and therefore better suited for less experienced operators. Direct insertion is more rapid, but it carries a greater risk. The tube may deviate somewhat from the intended line, and so the renal collecting system should be well dilated. This procedure is reserved for experienced operators.

A disposable, three-piece nephrostomy set has been developed for this technique. It is well suited for insertion under real-time ultrasound guidance but can be placed equally well under fluoroscopic vision. The drainage tube, which is available in a range of sizes, is easily exchanged if more permanent diversion is desired (e. g., during and after radiation therapy of gynecologic tumors).

The three-piece nephrostomy set (Angiomed, D-7505 Ettlingen) consists of a puncture needle, a rigid guide wire with a 6-cm soft flexible tip, and a pigtail drainage catheter (Fig. 70). The puncture needle possesses a central fine needle with stylet to allow optimum sonographic visualization of the needle tip. A discharge of urine from the needle confirms its location within the pyelocaliceal system and is very slight, so that the collecting system will remain sufficiently dilated for the manipulations that follow.

The rigid guide wire eliminates the tedious and painful process of developing a nephrostomy tract through the flank and renal capsule with plastic dilators. It forms a stable splint over which the catheter is effortlessly advanced with a rotary motion through the muscles and renal capsule to the desired position in the renal pelvis.

The nephrostomy is performed in three steps. Following three liberal skin preparations with merphene, sterile draping, and local anesthesia with 5–8 ml 1% lidocaine, the biopsy transducer is positioned over the posterolateral aspect of the kidney, as for a renal core biopsy.

The puncture needle is introduced through the central aperture of the transducer and through the skin (Fig. 71). The stylet is held in place with the index

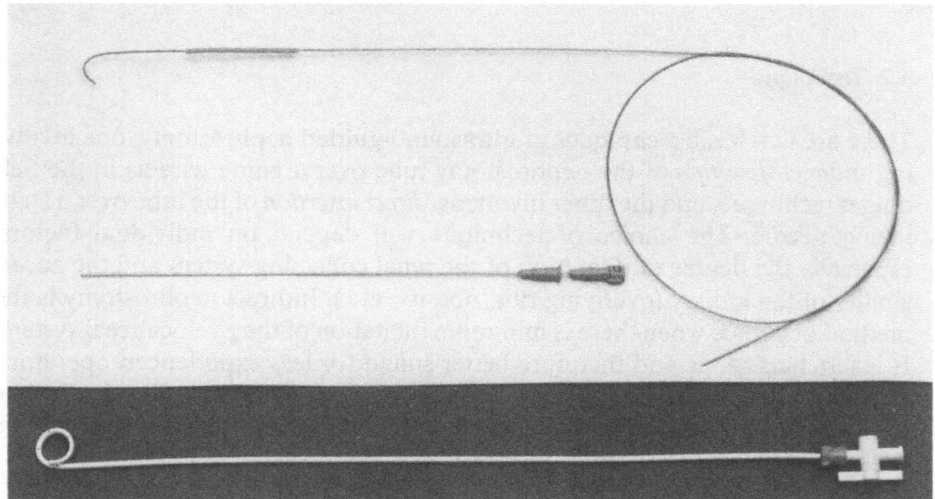

Fig. 70. Nephrostomy set 1: rigid guide wire with soft J tip *(top)*, initial puncture needle with central fine needle *(center)*, and pigtail drainage catheter *(bottom)*

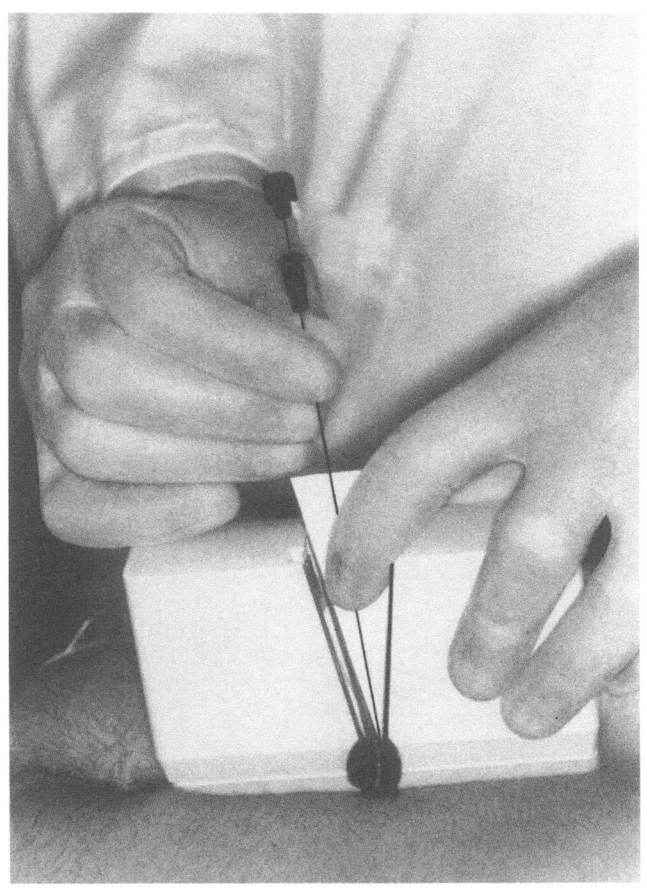

Fig. 71. The initial puncture needle is inserted into the skin and musculature through the biopsy transducer

finger just as in a fine-needle aspiration (Fig. 72). Within the renal pelvis the needle tip appears as a bright echo adjacent to the sight line (Fig. 73). The needle is advanced successively through the subcutaneous tissue, muscle, perirenal fat, renal capsule, and renal parenchyma. After the stylet is removed, a trickle of urine from the hub confirms correct placement within the renal pelvis.

Next the rigid guide wire is introduced through the puncture needle. A small plastic tube is used to help guide the soft, J-shaped tip of the wire into the bore of the needle (Fig. 74). As it leaves the needle and enters the collecting system, the tip of the wire will reassume its J shape and will be partly or completely visible depending on its position relative to the image plane (Fig. 75 a,b). The guide wire is fed through the needle until it engages against the opposite wall of the renal pelvis, and the rigid portion of the wire has penetrated the renal capsule and parenchyma (Fig. 76 a,b). With proper caution, there should be no

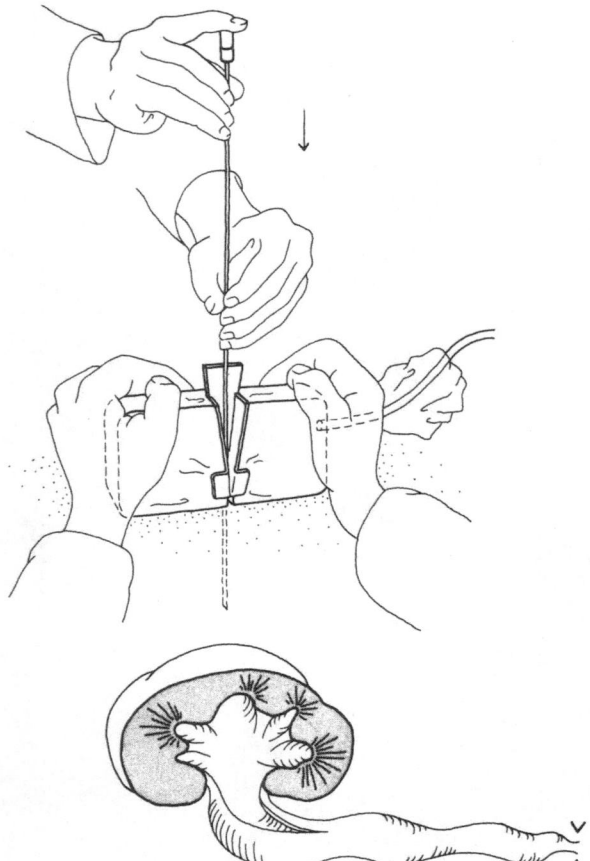

Fig. 72. The initial puncture needle is advanced through the skin, subcutaneous tissue, and muscle into the perirenal fat. Ordinarily, the needle is introduced at a slightly oblique angle (not shown here for reasons of perspective)

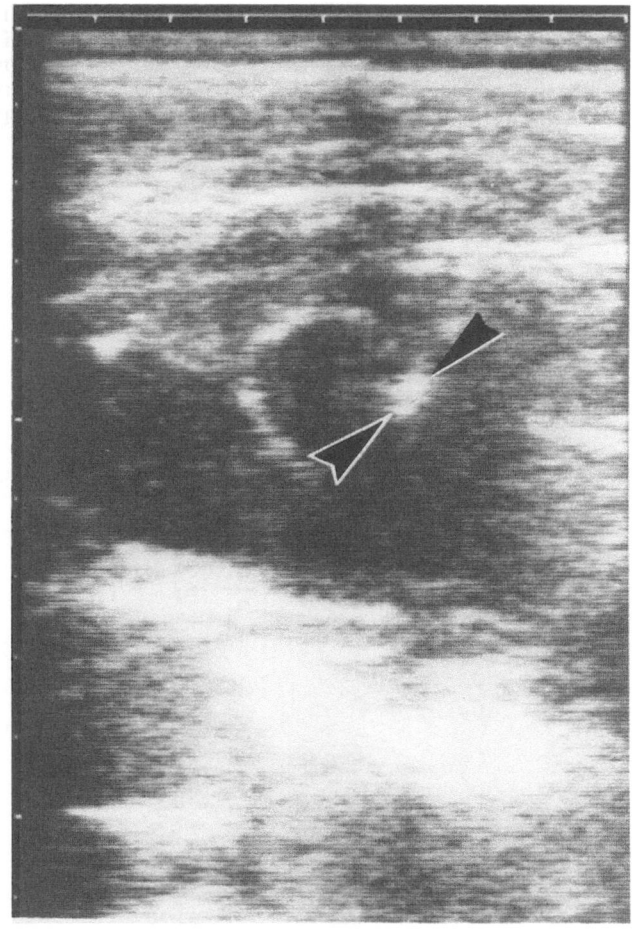

Fig. 73. The bright needle tip echo *(arrows)* is visualized by shifting the transducer slightly cranial, producing an apparent caudal shift of the puncture needle

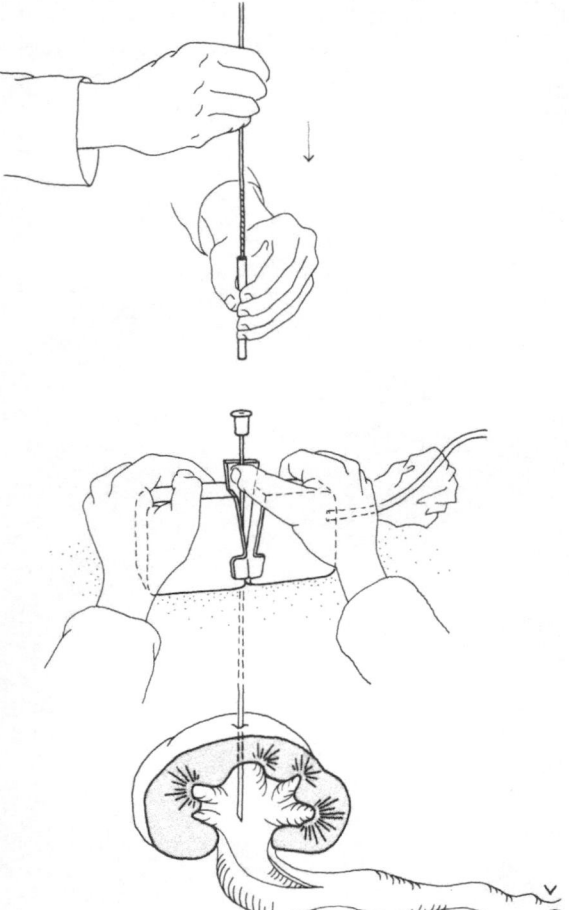

Fig. 74. The soft-tipped guide wire is introduced through the puncture needle. The soft, J-shaped tip is straightened by means of a short plastic tube to facilitate insertion

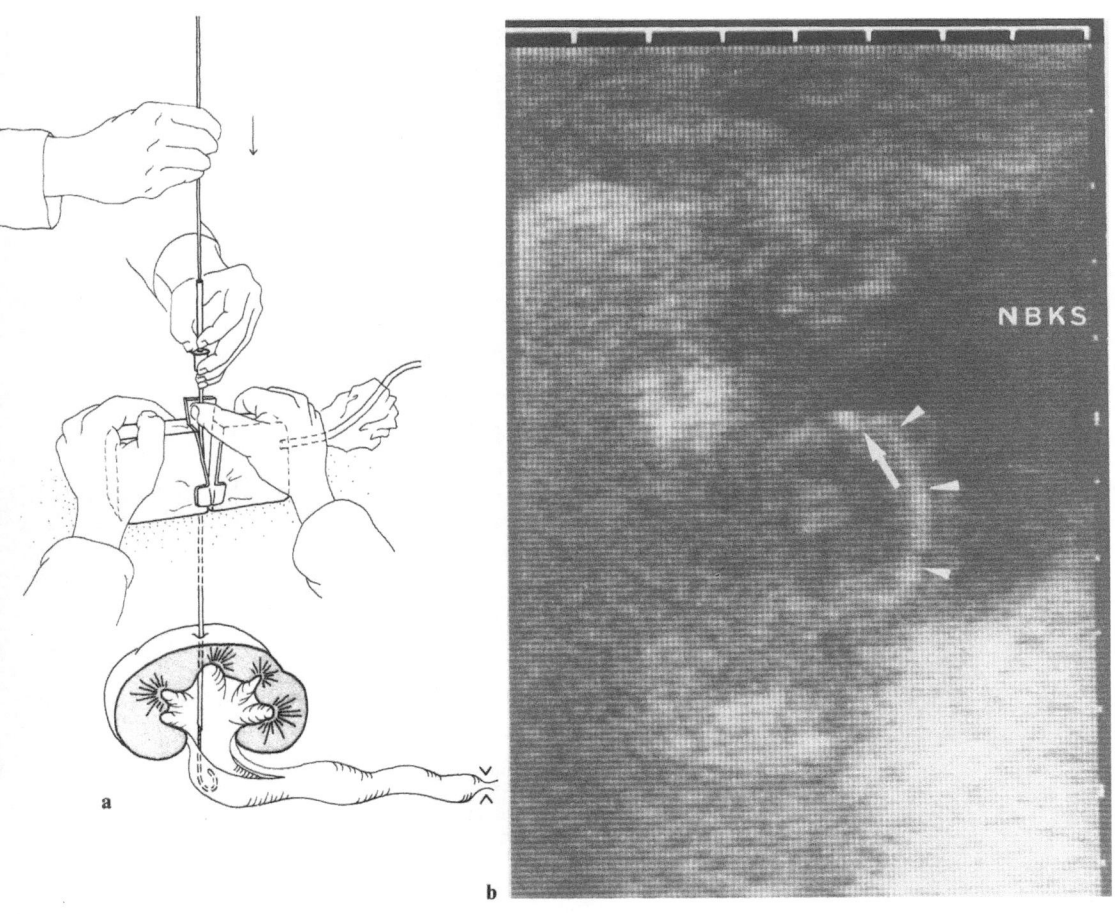

Fig. 75. a The soft tip of the rigid guide wire is visible in the renal pelvis and engages against its medial wall. **b** The curled tip of the wire is visible in the sonogram as an elliptical curve *(small arrows)*. The tip of the puncture needle *(large arrow)* is faintly visible

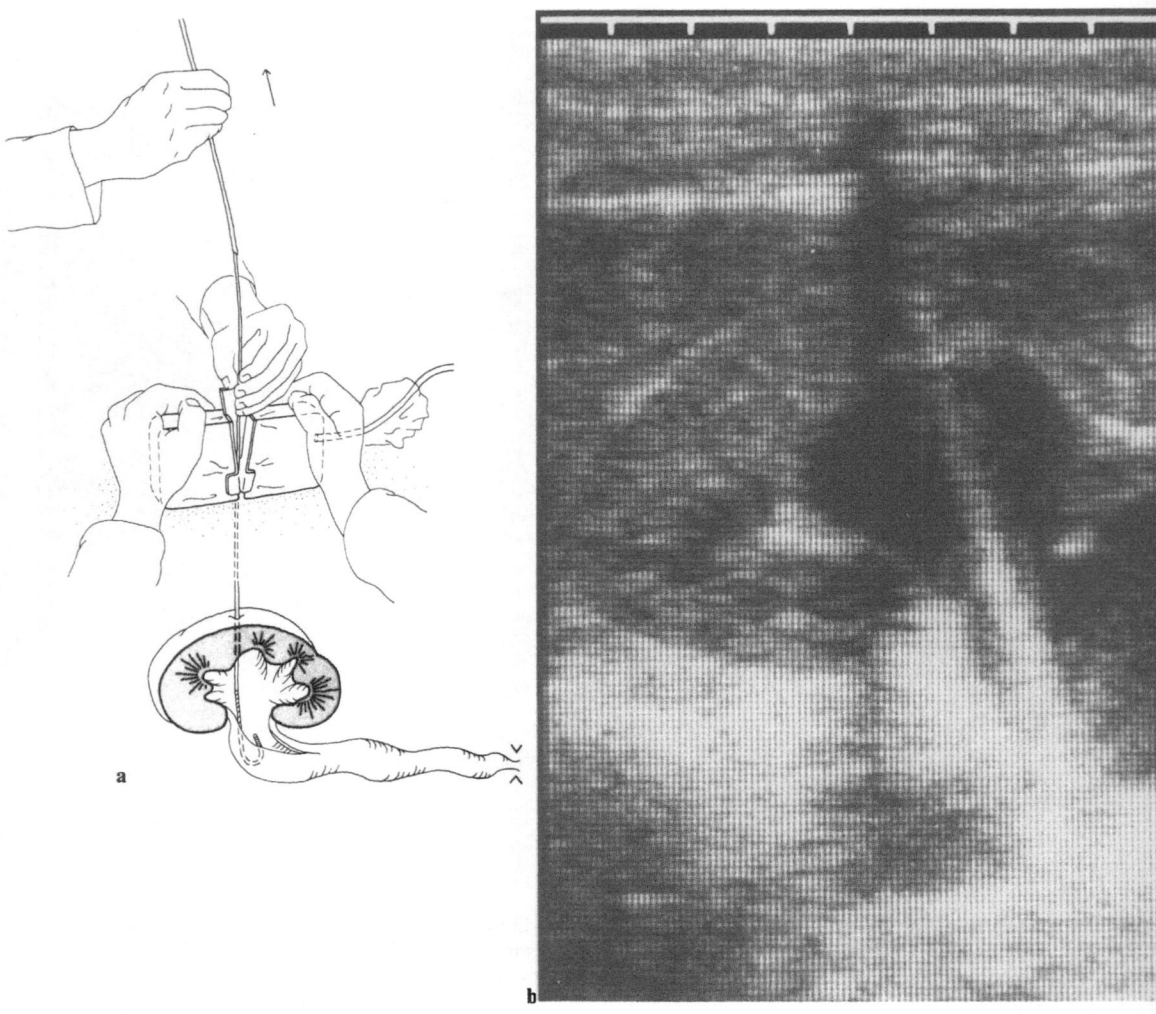

Fig. 76. a The soft tip of the guide wire is completely within the renal pelvis. The rigid part of the wire has likewise penetrated the renal capsule and pelvic wall. The puncture needle is removed. **b** Corresponding sonogram. The rigid part of the guide wire traverses the renal capsule and outer renal pelvic wall. The soft tip abuts on the anteromedial wall, and its curvature is apparent

danger of perforating the wall of the renal pelvis. Usually, the soft tip of the wire will slip down into the ureter.

Now the puncture needle is removed, taking strict care not to disturb the position of the guide wire. Finally, only the guide wire remains in the renal pelvis. The respiratory swing of the exposed part of the wire should be apparent at this time. Next a small skin incision is made along the guide wire, and the nephrostomy tube is advanced over the guide wire into the renal collecting system (Fig. 77). Again, care is taken not to displace the guide wire at this stage or push

130

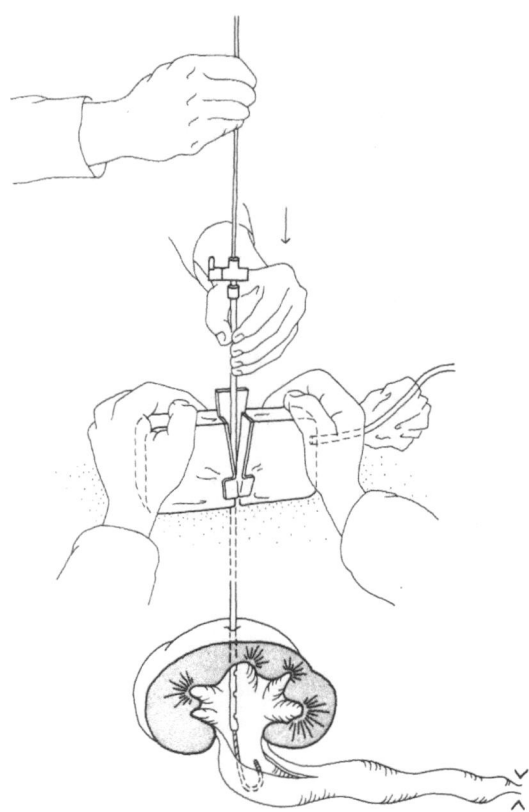

Fig. 77. The nephrostomy tube is advanced over the guide wire into the renal pelvis

its rigid portion deeper into the kidney. When the pigtail catheter is visible within the renal pelvis, the guide wire may be removed. All this is done under continuous sonographic vision.

The free flow of urine from the catheter confirms its correct placement. If the renal pelvis is no longer pressurized, or if its contents are highly viscous (pyonephrosis), the pelvis is aspirated with a syringe.

Proper placement of the nephrostomy tube is documented roentgenographically by injecting a low volume and a high volume of contrast medium through the catheter into the pyelocaliceal system (Fig. 78). Tube placement is adjusted as needed before the tube is secured to the skin. The rigid guide wire may be reintroduced to facilitate adjustments.

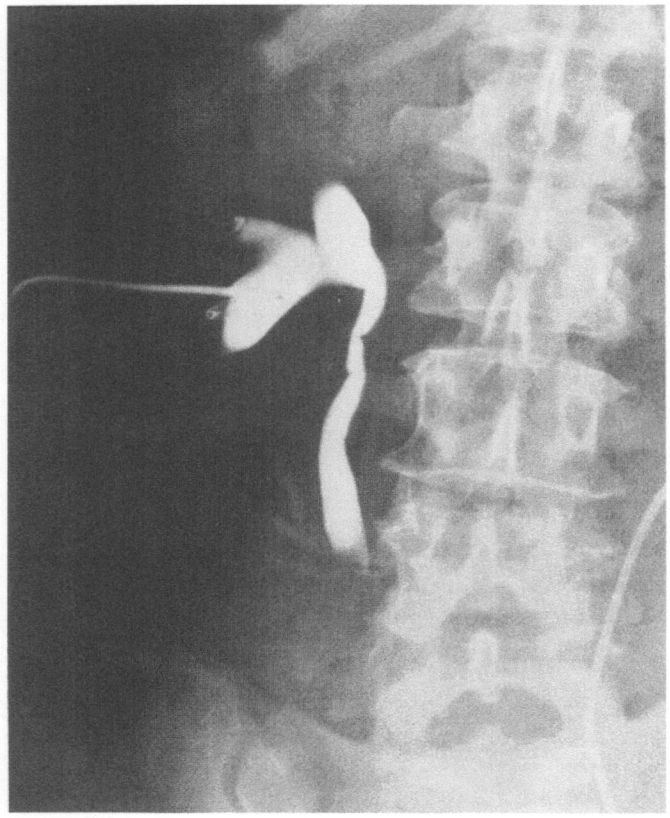

Fig. 78. Roentgenogram of the nephrostomy tube seated in the right renal pelvis. The peripheral urinary obstruction is caused by a low-lying bladder carcinoma

Percutaneous Transhepatic Chlangiography Principle

If the collecting system is sufficiently dilated and can be well delineated with ultrasound, it is possible to insert the nephrostomy tube directly into the kidney over a guide needle. This technique is similar to that formerly used for percutaneous transhepatic cholangiography. The drainage system is introduced through a small stab incision in the skin until the tip of the needle or catheter is within the subcutaneous tissue (Fig. 79). The centrally open transducer is moved into position around the catheter, and the sight line is positioned over the area of the renal pelvis that is to be punctured. The nephrostomy tube and guide needle are then advanced together along the sight line to the target (Fig. 80). Respiration is suspended during this phase. The muscles usually offer a tense, elastic resistance that is easily overcome.

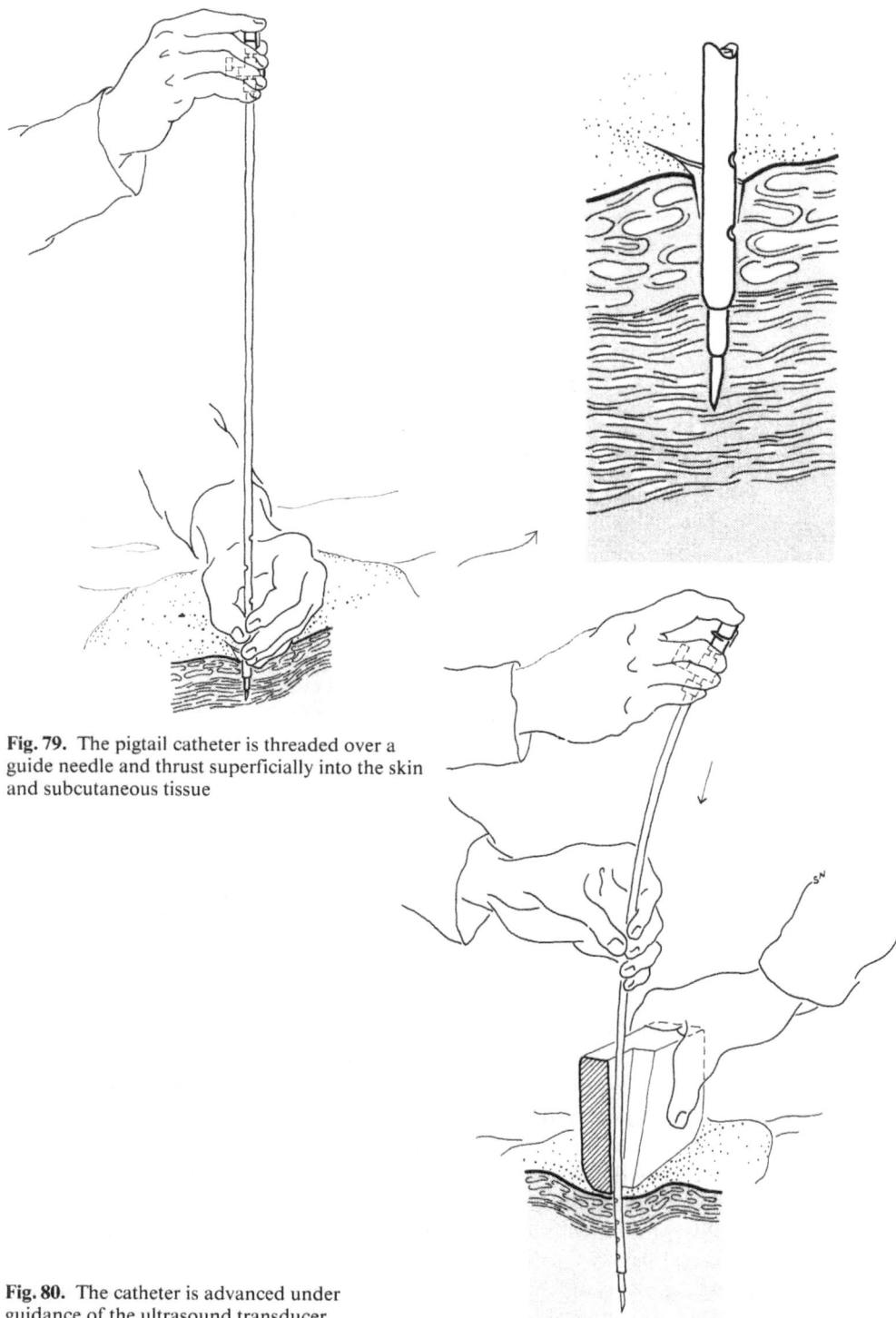

Fig. 79. The pigtail catheter is threaded over a guide needle and thrust superficially into the skin and subcutaneous tissue

Fig. 80. The catheter is advanced under guidance of the ultrasound transducer

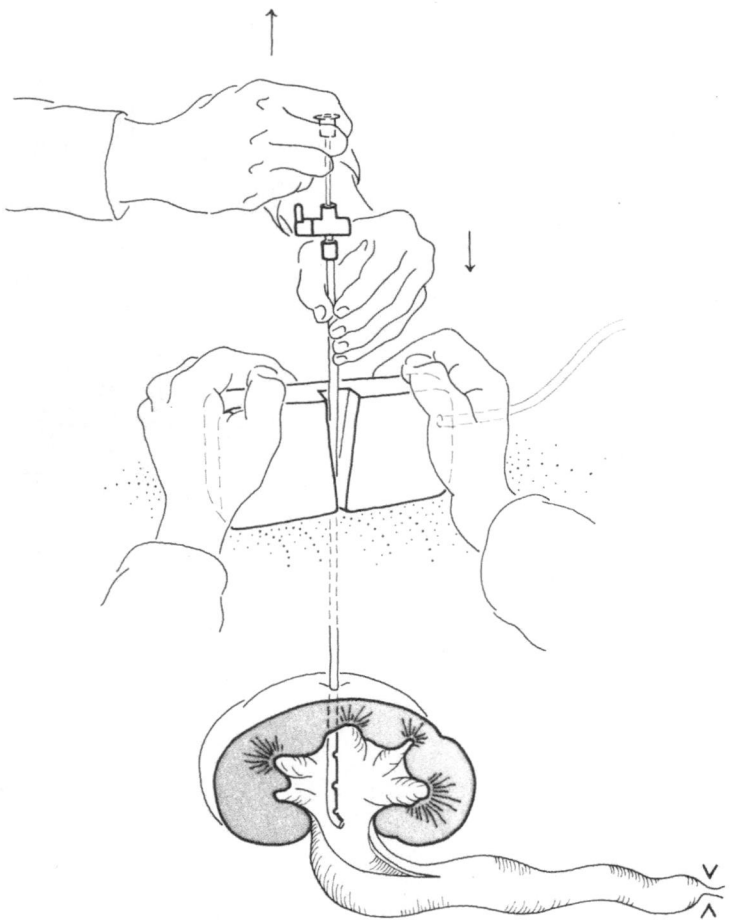

Fig. 81. a When the pigtail catheter has entered the renal pelvis, the guide needle is retracted somewhat while the catheter is simultaneously advanced. **b** Detail of the catheter tip during retraction of the needle

When the needle tip and catheter have reached the collecting system, the catheter is carefully pushed forward while the needle is simultaneously retracted (Fig. 81 a,b). A coiling movement of the pigtail catheter is clearly visible as the needle is withdrawn, and the catheter is advanced a short distance farther until the coil appears to be optimally positioned within the renal pelvis (Fig. 82). This is confirmed by the discharge of urine on removal of the needle.

If the collecting system is not pressurized or if pyonephrosis exists, the renal pelvis must be aspirated with a syringe to determine whether satisfactory drainage has been established.

Again, roentgenograms are taken with a low volume and high volume of contrast medium injected (Fig. 83) to confirm correct tube placement. Ante-

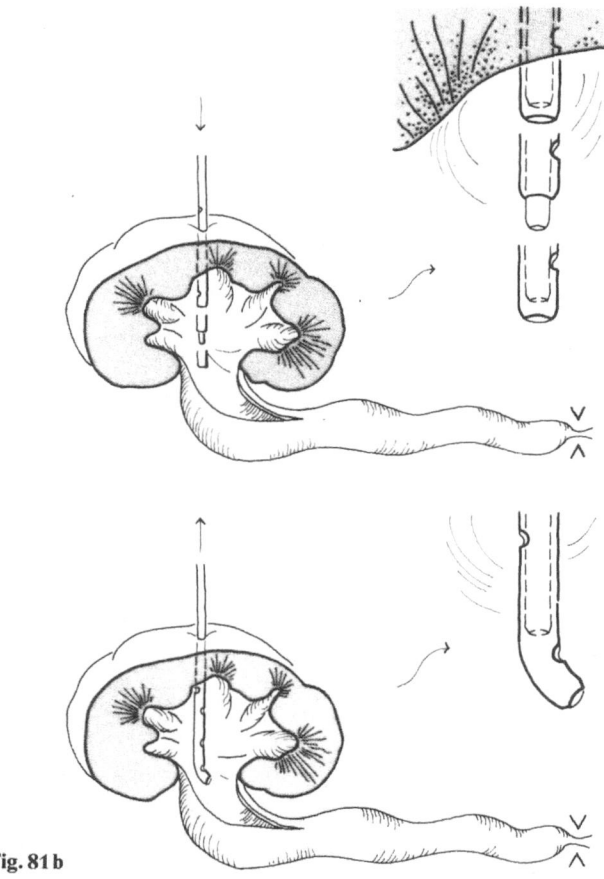

Fig. 81 b

grade pyelograms may be obtained at this time to establish the cause of the peripheral obstruction if it is not already known.

Occasionally, a bilateral nephrostomy is necessary. The surgical technique is analogous, and both nephrostomies may be performed at the same sitting. The choice of nephrostomy set and insertion method will depend entirely on individual circumstances and the accessibility of the renal pelvis. Occasionally, we have passed a catheter/needle combination directly into a grossly dilated renal pelvis on one side, while using the Seldinger technique to catheterize a minimally dilated collecting system on the opposite side. Of course, all nephrostomies are performed under real-time ultrasound guidance.

As a rule, supervision after percutaneous nephrostomy consists of fluoroscopy with injection of contrast material and sonography to evaluate the area around the punctured kidney. Computed tomography is occasionally useful as an adjunct. This is illustrated by the following case.

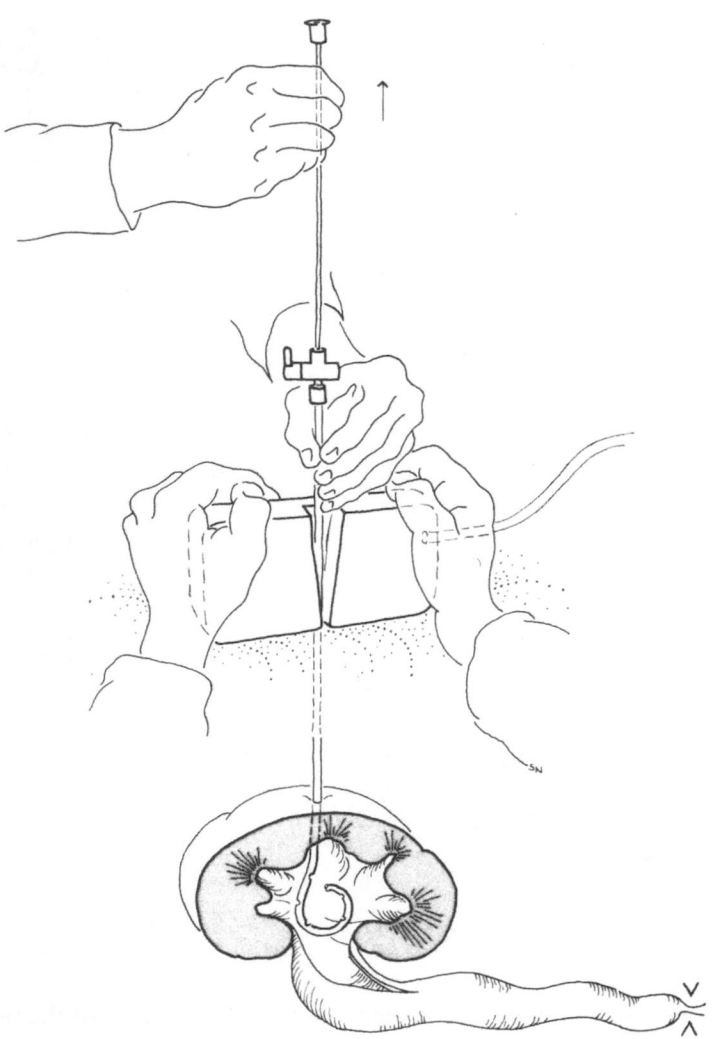

Fig. 82. When the tip has assumed its coiled shape, it can be manipulated into the desired position with the guide needle

A 52-year-old woman had undergone radiation therapy for a massive gynecologic tumor, resulting in total occlusion of the left ureter. Initially, a left percutaneous nephrostomy was performed (Fig. 84). The ureter was obstructed distally by the tumor. A computed tomographic scan made several days later showed small, nodular, juxtaaortic masses on the left side that were consistent

136

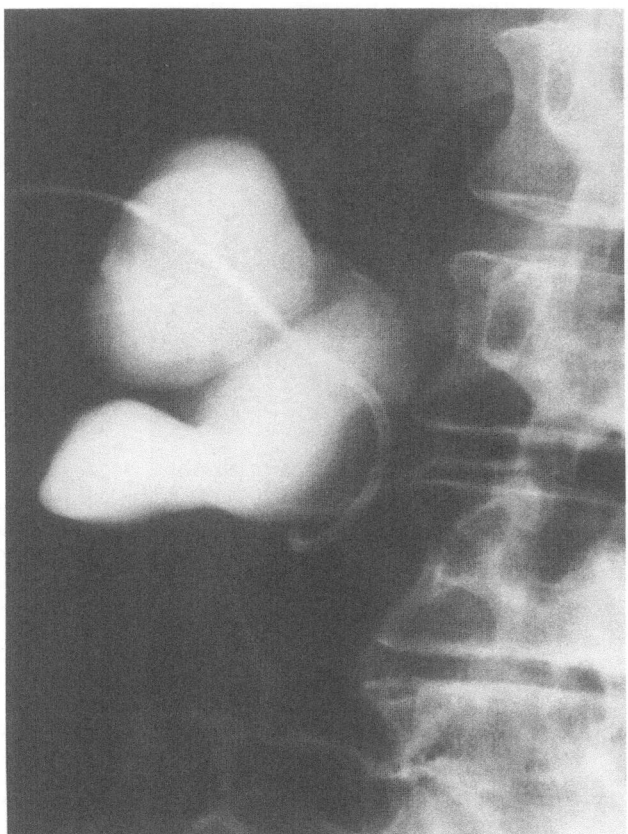

Fig. 83. A pigtail nephrostomy catheter is introduced into the grossly dilated right renal pelvis using the percutaneos transhepatic cholangiography technique; there is a ureteropelvic stenosis of vascular etiology

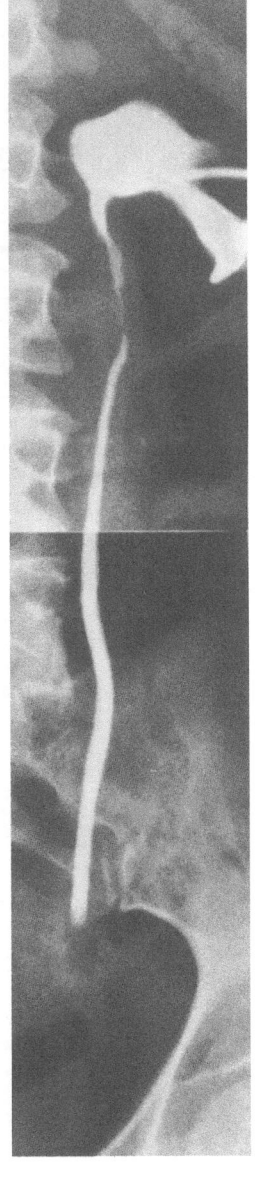

Fig. 84. Obstruction of the left upper urinary tract by a massive ▷ gynecologic tumor in the lesser pelvis. A nephrostomy was performed under ultrasound guidance. There is no drainage of contrast material into the bladder

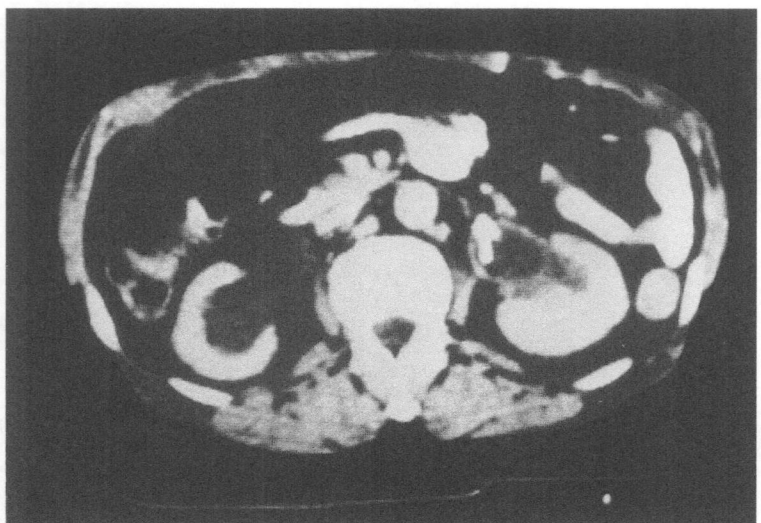

Fig. 85. Same patient as in Fig. 84. A computed tomographic scan obtained several days later shows another urinary obstruction on the right side. Small, nodular lesions adjacent to the aorta are suggestive of metastasis. On the left side the nephrostomy catheter is visible in the mildly dilated renal pelvis

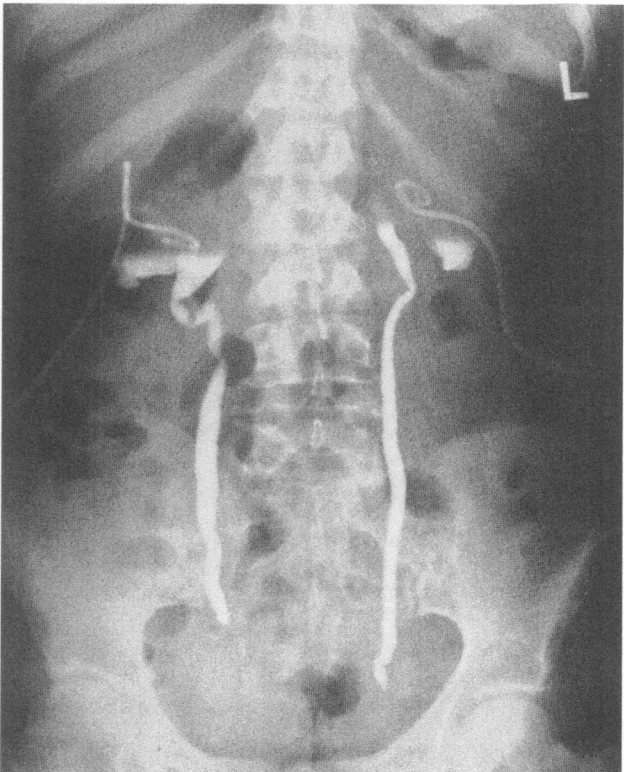

Fig. 86. Same patient as in Fig. 85, 2 weeks later. A second nephrostomy has been performed on the right side. The size of the tumor in the lesser pelvis can be appreciated from the course of the contrast-filled ureters (patient in upright position)

with lymph node metastases (Fig. 85). The scan demonstrates the nephrostomy tube in the left renal pelvis, which is still dilated. Before long a second percutaneous nephrostomy had to be performed on the right side (Fig. 86). The urinary obstruction by the tumor in the lesser pelvis is now clearly visible on both sides.

3.3 Drainage Catheters: Materials and Selection

Owing to the development of new technologies, percutaneous nephrostomy has become a rapid and low-risk therapeutic measure. With ultrasound, it is possible to pass drainage tubes percutaneously into the renal pelvis with great accuracy via the most direct route available.

The new nephrostomy sets have proved excellent for this procedure. The polymeric material used for the nephrostomy tubes contributes significantly to the long-term success of the drainage. *Polyurethane* can be manufactured in a range of flexibilities and is an excellent material for internal stents because it is soft yet, in contrast to silicone, is not susceptible to collapse. The tendency of polyurethane to retain its original shape is disadvantageous for percutaneous diversion, however, because the catheter is not flexible enough to follow organ movements.

We have found *polyethylene* to be a superior material for percutaneous drainage catheters, and we use it exclusively. This material has excellent gliding properties and wall stability and, like polyurethane, is resistant to encrustation. The material must be appropriately surface-treated, and materials of this type are offered by various manufacturers in a range of qualities. The resistance of a material to encrustation can be accurately assessed on the basis of struvite deposits observed with the polarizing microscope [65]. Clinical experience confirms the excellent encrustation resistance of our percutaneous nephrostomy catheters, which in many cases may be left indwelling for months or even years without loss of patency.

The relative stiffness of the catheter material at room temperature facilitates its passage into the renal pelvis or into an abscess cavity. At body temperature it becomes softer and more pliable, which makes prolonged use of the tube easier to tolerate and reduces skin irritation around the nephrostomy site. We have observed no instances of catheter breakage.

Percutaneous nephrostomy offers a significant advantage to both the patient and physician: the patient himself can check for adequate drainage function at any time without the need for auxiliary instruments.

The placement of ureteral stent catheters has become a frequent and routine procedure [48, 56, 106]. For the patient, it is initially more invasive, sometimes presents difficulties, and requires regular supervision after placement. If percutaneous diversion is maintained after the antegrade insertion of a stent catheter, the stent should only be used temporarily [54]. However, internal drainage via an indwelling ureteral stent may be maintained permanently in selected cases [62].

The use of ultrasound guidance for percutaneous nephrostomy is undoubtedly a great advantage for the physician and patient and is more important than the choice of a particular nephrostomy set. Nevertheless, roentgenography cannot be entirely dispensed with in these patients, especially when one considers the value of contrast films in documenting the position of the drain and of antegrade pyelograms in establishing the cause of the obstruction.

A swift, smooth placement of the nephrostomy tube is important in terms of patient acceptance, and it reduces the risk of faulty insertion and other complications. The suitability of the different nephrostomy sets for ultrasound guidance varies, and so they should be individually adapted as required.

Set 1 (for the Seldinger technique) is the most foolproof and is best suited for physicians who have had little experience with the method (see Fig. 70, p. 124). This set is preferred for the puncture of a minimally dilated renal pelvis, or for establishing drainage of biliary passages in patients with obstructive jaundice, for example.

Set 2 (for simultaneous insertion of the needle and nephrostomy tube; Angiomed, D-7505 Ettlingen) is advantageous when the collecting system is well dilated. The drainage system can be passed into the renal pelvis in seconds under ultrasound guidance, and the catheter tip will immediately assume the desired pigtail shape when the guide needle is withdrawn (Fig. 82). This set is equally well suited for abscess drainage or for the palliative diversion of a pleural effusion or ascites.

Set 3 is a special modification of set 2 [149] that is appropriate for any degree of pyelocaliceal dilatation, because it allows a low-risk "exploratory" puncture to be made. In other respects the set utilizes the basic principle of set 1, in that a rigid needle is introduced initially to serve as a guide for advancing the flexible drainage catheter through the soft renal capsule. This avoids the necessity of using dilators to make a nephrostomy tract in cases where there is little back pressure in the renal pelvis.

Given the high accuracy and safety of percutaneous nephrostomy under sonographic guidance, the procedure may be elected at a relatively early stage, before an impending deterioration of renal function becomes manifest. The method also has value in the modern techniques of anatrophic nephrolithotomy and extracorporeal shock-wave lithotripsy.

Therapeutic percutaneous nephrostomy is particularly appropriate in cases where only one kidney is obstructed by tumor, for example, and demonstrates hydronephrotic change [57].

In patients with stone disease and progressive uremia, the percutaneous diversion of only one kidney often affords marked and rapid clinical improvement with a normalization of creatinine values. The resulting diuresis produces an irrigating effect that may assist the passage even of large stones, making them accessible to extraction with the Zeiss loop. In these cases nephrostomy should not be delayed.

It is reasonable to expect that the rapid development of percutaneous lithotripsy will also expand the role of percutaneous nephrostomy. In addition, the procedure is likely to gain importance as an adjunct to extracorporeal shock-wave lithotripsy as utilization of that therapy increases.

3.4 The Loop Catheter

Fixation of the drainage tube to the skin remains a difficult problem. A suture would seem to be the most logical means of securing the tube. This conforms to general surgical opinion, but it is not entirely satisfactory. The relatively smooth drainage tube can easily slip out of the suture loop if the suture has been loosened by wound discharges. During abscess drainage, moreover, an inflammatory skin reaction soon develops around the tube, and the skin is unable to retain the stitch.

Various methods of securing the drain have been considered in an effort to circumvent this problem. The most popular device has been the self-retaining balloon catheter, but serious problems have occurred during the everyday use of this device (decubitus, excessive traction with rupture of kidney, etc.).

We have found that the pigtail loop catheter provides a very secure, internal retention at low risk. A loop of thin nylon thread extends from the tip of the

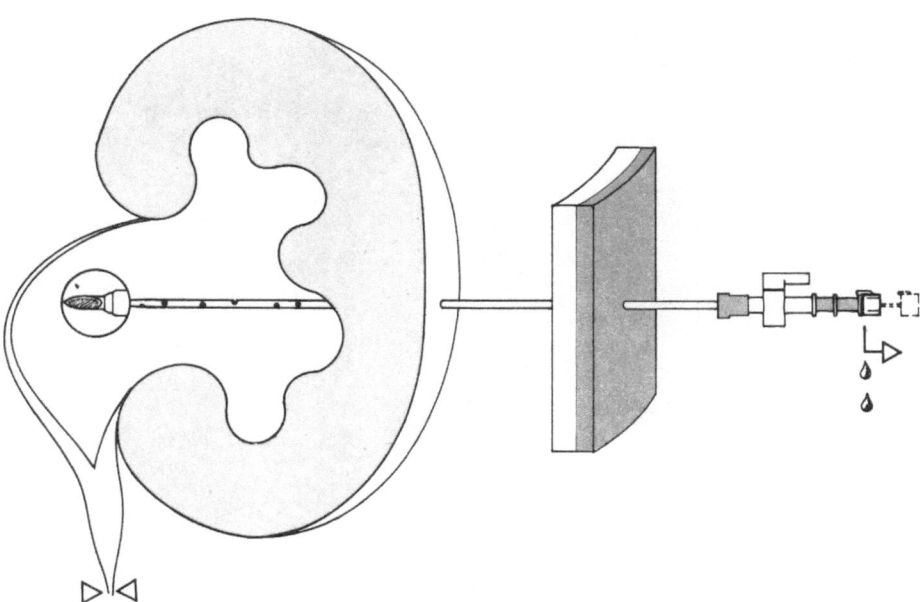

Fig. 87. Nephrostomy set 2. The pigtail catheter is straightened with the aid of the catheter straightener and replaced with the nested puncture needles. The internal stylet is for confirming correct placement by the aspiration of urine *(arrow)*

141

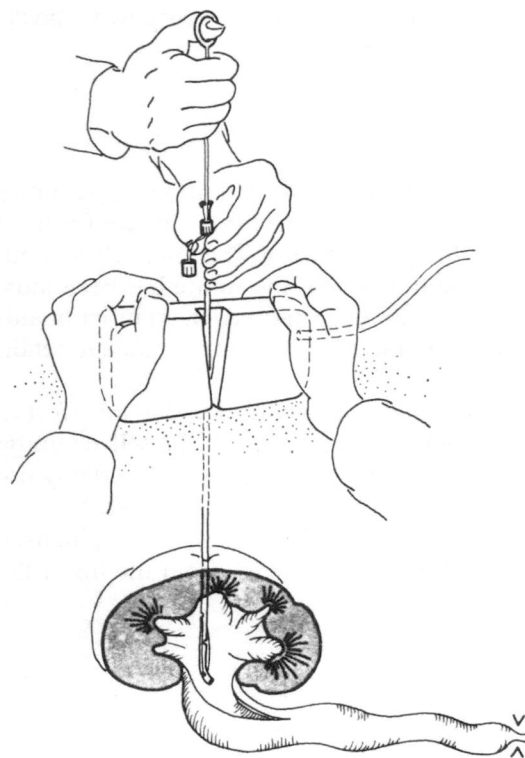

Fig. 88. The nephrostomy tube with central guide needle is inserted through the tissue into the kidney. The nylon thread lies flat against the distal end of the tube. When the guide needle is withdrawn, the catheter tip will assume its original pigtail shape

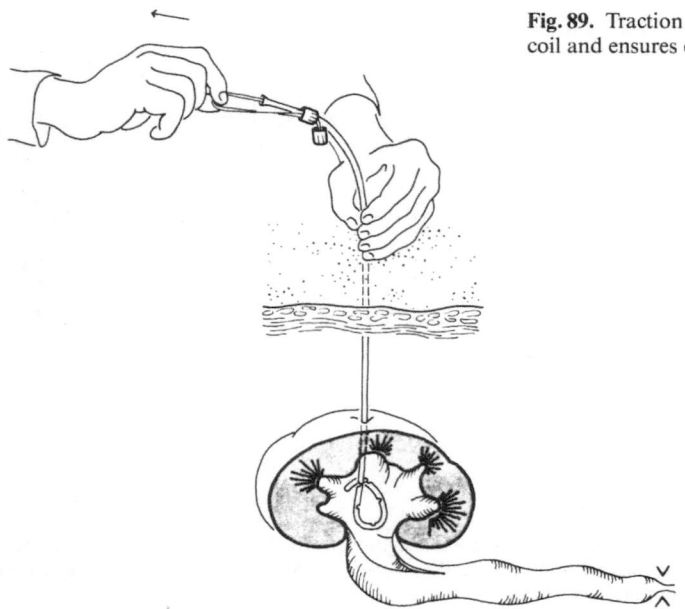

Fig. 89. Traction on the thread secures the coil and ensures catheter retention

catheter to its external end, where it can be anchored with a screw fastener. This makes it possible to secure the pigtail shape of the catheter tip and thus protect the catheter from inadvertent dislodgement.

The tube is introduced using the direct nephrostomy technique. The pigtail catheter is first threaded over the guide needle, and this assembly is inserted into the renal pelvis. The thin nylon thread lies closely against the surface of the catheter and does not interfere with the insertion (Fig. 88). After removal of the guide needle, the thread can be pulled tight at the catheter tip (Fig. 89). Before this, during retraction of the needle, the pigtail catheter is advanced a short distance farther until it is centrally positioned within the collecting system and can spontaneously assume its original coiled shape. Finally, the coil is secured with the nylon thread. This arrangement provides very good urinary diversion while ensuring self-retention of the catheter within the kidney.

Case Report:

A woman born in 1919, who was known to have chronic pyelonephritis and multiple parenchymal calcifications but showed no evidence of medullary sponge kidney, suffered febrile episodes and had a markedly elevated sedimentation rate. She had a long history of phenacetin abuse. At presentation a neoplastic disorder was suspected. An excretory urogram showed bilaterally shrunken kidneys with parenchymal calcifications and an absence of excretion on the right side. Sonography showed marked dilatation of the renal collecting system. Retrograde filling was attempted but was unsuccessful because of an obstruction in the distal third of the ureter (Fig. 90 a-c).

In view of the right urinary obstruction and bouts of septic fever, right pyonephrosis was presumed, and an ultrasound-guided percutaneous nephrostomy was ordered. When the pigtail catheter was passed into the renal pelvis and contrast medium was instilled, gross dilatation of the collecting system and ureter became apparent. A small shadow was noted in the distal third of the ureter, consistent with a ureteral stone (Fig. 90 b). When the patient was brought to the standing position, a small amount of contrast medium drained into the bladder. A narrow stenosis in the distal ureter was demonstrated, as well as masses of debris in the dilated midportion of the ureter and peripheral, circular lucencies consistent with cystic ureteritis (Fig. 90 c).

After the procedure, renal function improved rapidly and the patient is temperature returned to normal. Use of the loop catheter avoided the problem of skin infection at the nephrostomy site.

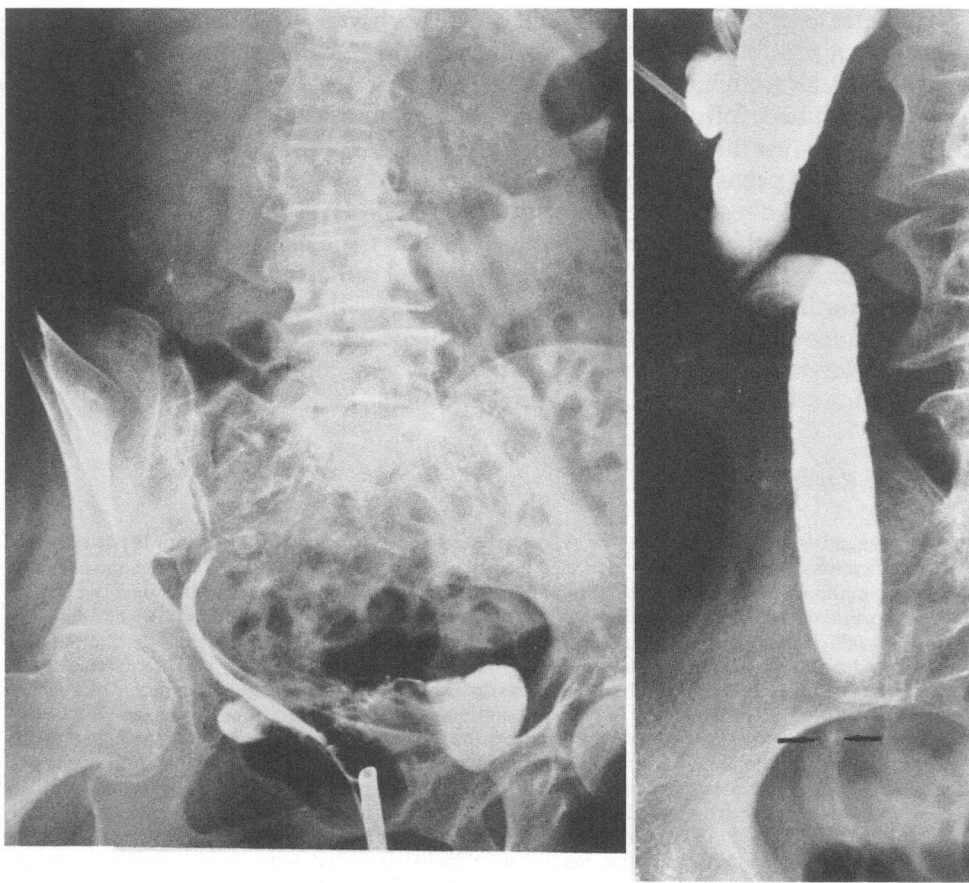

a

Fig. 90 a-c. Bilaterally shrunken kidneys with parenchymal calcifications. **a** Retrograde urogram of the right side. Contrast flow is halted by an obstruction in the distal ureter. Radiolucent stone? Sloughed papilla? **b** Antegrade urogram via the percutaneous nephrostomy. Note the marked dilatation of the pyelocaliceal system and ureter and the obstructing stone in the distal third of the ureter *(arrows)*. **c** Exposure with patient in standing position shows some drainage of contrast medium into the bladder. A narrow stenosis is evident in the distal third of the ureter, and there is cystic ureteritis in the middle third with debris

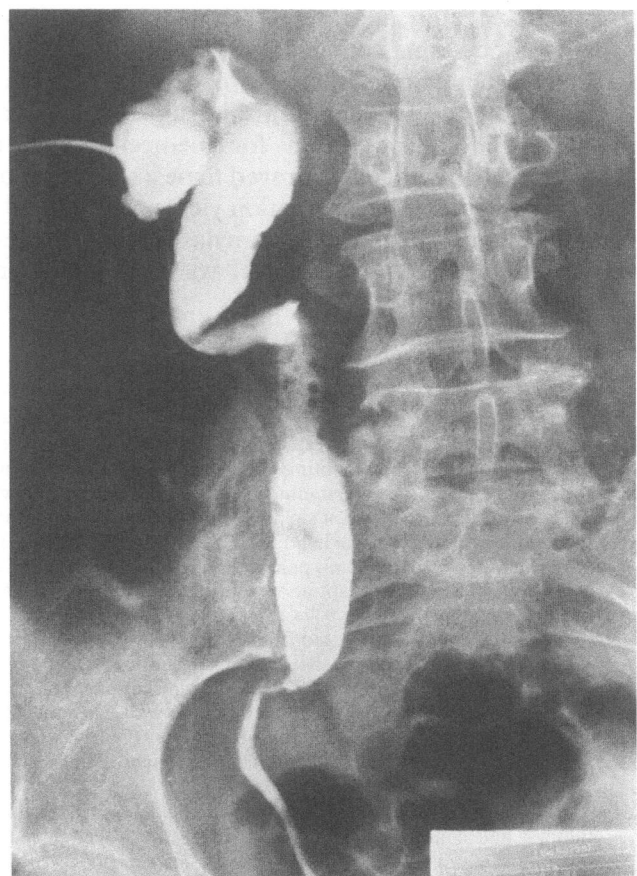

Fig. 90 c

4 Aspiration of Pancreatic Pseudocysts

The pancreatic pseudocyst is a typical complication of chronic pancreatitis. Although many pseudocysts resolve spontaneously, operative removal is frequently necessary and generally consists of marsupialization, extirpation, or partial pancreatic resection. Formerly, very large pseudocysts were also treated by external drainage. However, this method had a high association with fistulous tract formation and other complications, and it was abandoned as operative treatment techniques improved.

When ultrasound is used to investigate pancreatic disease, one frequently encounters space-occupying lesions whose benignancy or malignancy is indeterminate, and which cannot be further differentiated by ultrasound alone. A

145

hypoechoic feature may represent a neoplasm, well-perfused edematous tissue, or a pseudocyst that contains debris.

When sonographic findings are inconclusive, fine-needle aspiration cytology can be of great value in furnishing a pathologic diagnosis. A number of patients have been referred to us for fine-needle aspirations in whom an initially unidentified growth lesion proved to be a small pseudocyst. This diagnosis was grossly presumed when aspiration yielded a clear and watery or slightly hemorrhagic fluid that showed a high amylase content in the laboratory. In these cases ultrasound-guided puncture can have occasional therapeutic as well as definitive diagnostic value.

Case Report:

A 40-year-old man had suffered attacks of pancreatitis for 4½ years. He experienced a renewed exacerbation with intractable vomiting. At hospitalization, sonograms showed an enlarged pancreas that appeared edematous and sonolucent; two small pseudocysts were demonstrated.

Eight weeks later the patient's clinical condition had deteriorated somewhat. Scans revealed a 3-cm pseudocyst located in the head of the pancreas (Fig. 91 a-e). Because clinical evidence of biliary obstruction, emaciation, and pain radiating to the back raised the possibility of malignant disease, an ultrasound-guided aspiration biopsy was performed. The aspiration yielded 10 ml of a slightly hemorrhagic fluid (Fig. 91 b, c). Afterward the pseudocyst could no longer be demonstrated. The amylase level in the aspirated fluid was 54000 U/l; cytology disclosed the presence of foam cells, leukocytes, and debris consistent with a pseudocyst that had undergone inflammatory change.

A roentgenogram taken after the injection of contrast material into the aspirated pseudocyst (about 3 ml, diluted) demonstrated a smooth cyst wall that showed a few small, pointed extensions and did not communicate with the pancreatic duct (Fig. 91 d). The contrast film definitely excluded the possibility of a choledochal diverticulum, which had been considered by the referring physician.

Repeat sonograms 4 months later confirmed the improved sonolucency of the entire gland. The pseudocyst had completely regressed. Circumscribed echoes in the head of the pancreas represented multiple small, necrotic zones showing evidence of calcification (Fig. 91 e).

This case illustrates that a small but symptomatic pancreatic pseudocyst can respond well to percutaneous treatment. This revives an earlier surgical treatment concept that is somewhat difficult to reconcile with present-day treatment modalities.

Given the small numbers of patients who have been treated by this method to date, it is still too early to decide whether the diagnostic procedure of aspiration cytology for pancreatic masses can have therapeutic value in selected cases. This question must be resolved in a larger patient population and over a longer period of time.

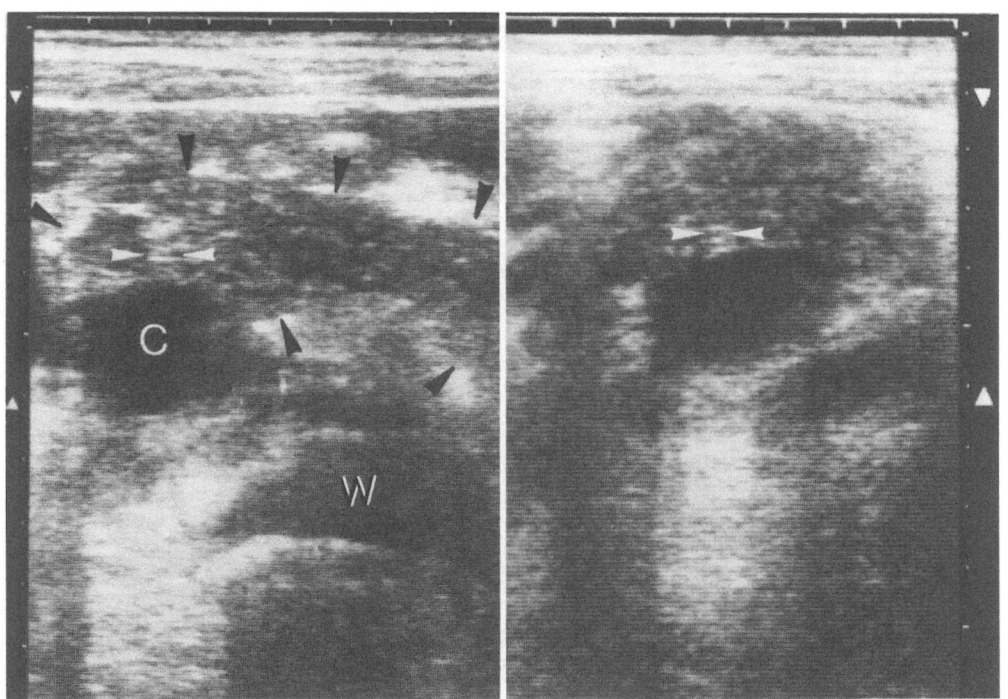

Fig. 91 a-e. Pancreatic pseudocyst.
a Transverse scan through the edematous pancreas *(black arrows)*. A pseudocyst *(C)* is demonstrated in the head of the pancreas. The pancreatic duct is marked with *white arrows. W,* spine. **b** Longitudinal scan through the enlarged head of the pancreas, again documenting the pseudocyst located posterior to the pancreatic duct *(arrows)*. **c** Longitudinal scan at same site as in Fig. 91 b The aspiration needle (tip marked with *arrow)* is within the pseudocyst, which is almost completely drained. **d** Pseudocyst drained by fine-needle aspiration and partially filled with contrast material. There is no extravasation and no communication with the pancreatic duct. **e** Follow-up sonogram taken 6 weeks after ultrasound-guided drainage of the pancreatic pseudocyst. The pseudocyst has not recurred. There is still residual pancreatic edema *(arrows)*, and small (calcifying?) necrotic foci are visible in the head of the pancreas

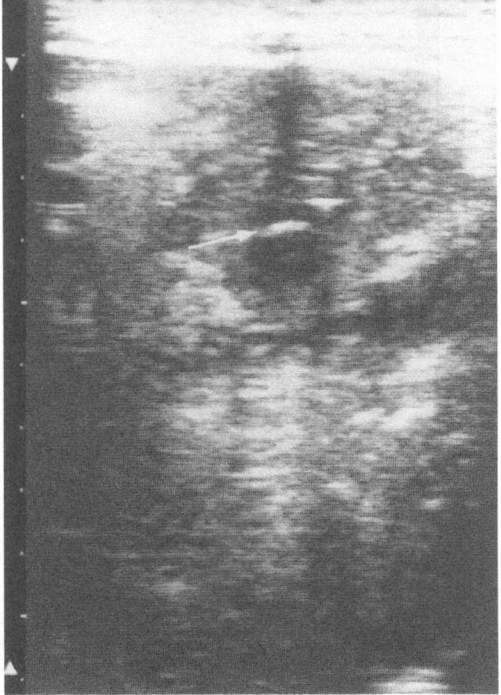

c

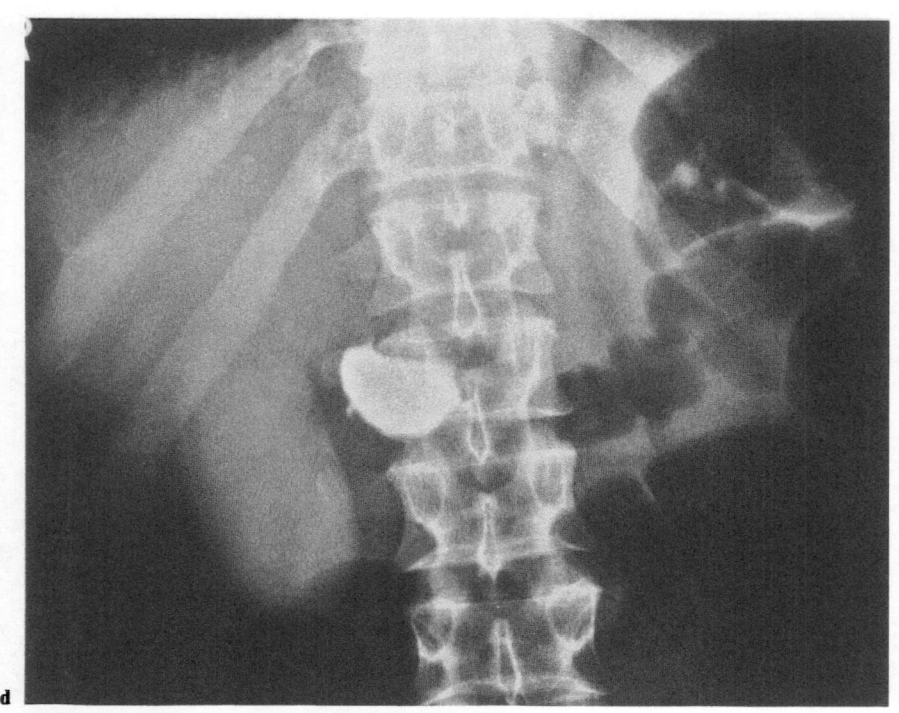

d

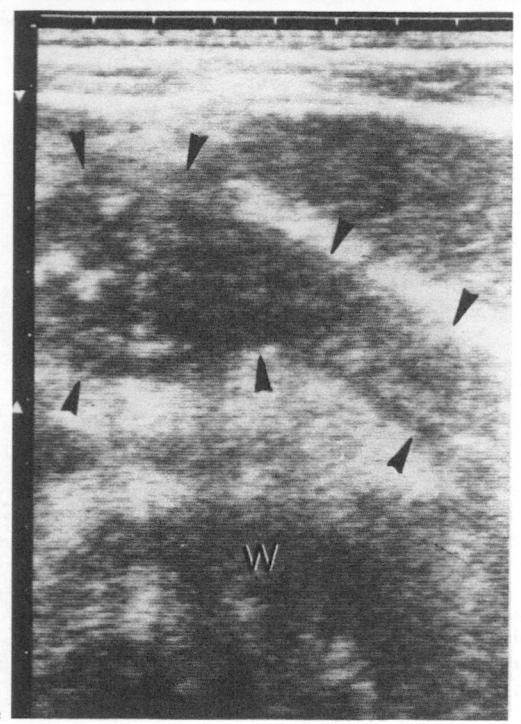

e

E. Concluding Remarks

Ultrasound-guided procedures at our center have established themselves within a short time as an important and even indispensable adjunct to sonography. In many cases the selective acquisition of tissue samples is necessary in order to confirm a macromorphological diagnosis, distinguish benign from malignant lesions, establish a prognosis, and accurately evaluate a previously detected focal anomaly in an organ. Often the results of these basic examinations – cross-sectional imaging and aspiration cytology – must be known before definitive therapy can be planned. An accurate diagnosis relies on the availability of a competent and well-equipped cytology laboratory staffed by trained experts who are experienced enough to classify and evaluate cellular material with a high degree of accuracy.

In some cases, however, cytologic examinations are unable to establish the nature of an organic lesion. In these cases an ultrasound-guided needle biopsy may be used to obtain histologic specimens (liver, kidney). This involves a somewhat higher risk because the procedure is necessarily more traumatizing to tissues. In this regard the newly developed thin cutting-edge needle represents a rational compromise between the fine cytology needle and conventional large-caliber biopsy needles. Occasionally, it can provide a more accurate evaluation of tumors that are not readily identifiable with aspiration cytology (lymphoma, hepatoma, etc.).

The risk of complications from needle punctures appears to be manageable when ultrasound guidance is used, as long as certain safety precautions are observed. Even so, the physician must understand that none of these procedures are entirely innocuous. In all cases the anticipated diagnostic benefit must be carefully weighed against the potential for harm. The puncture should be done only if it will contribute substantially to therapeutic decision making, and especially if it will obviate the need for further, more invasive measures (laparoscopy, operation, etc.).

Puncture techniques for the selective sampling of tissues have recently been joined by percutaneous methods of therapy. Besides percutaneous nephrostomy, percutaneous abscess drainage in particular has achieved clinical importance in appropriately selected cases. If successful, percutaneous abscess drainage can eliminate the need for operative measures (in up to 80% of cases); if unsuccessful, the option of operative treatment still remains.

Ultrasound guidance offers several advantages over guidance by computed tomography, with which it sometimes competes: It enables the very rapid insertion of biopsy needles and drainage catheters, it involves no radiation exposure, it furnishes dynamic information with real-time imaging, it allows continual bedside monitoring (e. g., for postbiopsy hemorrhage), and its costs are relatively low.

It is reasonable to expect that the use of ultrasound-guided fine-needle aspiration biopsies in particular will continue to develop and expand, for they are essential to the definitive diagnosis of organ lesions detected with ultrasound. The differential diagnosis of these lesions is too broad and complex to be effectively accomplished without benefit of cytologic analysis.

It remains to be seen how the development of new technologies (computer-assisted sonography, nuclear magnetic resonance imaging) will advance the field of noninvasive diagnosis. In the meantime, it is apparent that ultrasound- and computed-tomography-guided biopsies and microscopic tissue analysis will continue to play a major role due to cost considerations alone.

References

1. Ackermann LV, Wheat MW (1955) The implantation of cancer. An avoidable surgical risk? Surgery 37: 341
2. Akorbiantz A (1983) Diskussionsbeitrag. In: Symposium über „Aktuelle Probleme der Echinokokkose" der Schweiz. Arbeitsgruppe für Echinokokkose, Zürich (16.6. 1983)
3. Alfidi RJ, Haaga J, Meaney TF et al. (1975) Computed tomography of the thorax and abdomen; a preliminary report. Radiology 117: 257–264
4. Allen TW, Honeckman CC (1974) Subcutaneous metastasis following needle biopsy of the pleura. J Am Osteopathol Assoc 73: 522–525
5. Anderson JE (ed) (1976) Muir's textbook of pathology, 10th edn. Arnold, London
6. Bachmann HJ (1979) Komplikationen und Kontraindikationen von perkutaner und offener Nierenbiopsie bei Kindern. In: Olbing H (Hrsg) Nierenbiopsie bei Kindern. Springer, Berlin Heidelberg New York, S 69–78
7. Bahlmann J, Otto P (1972) Perkutane Nierenbiopsie mit Ultraschall-Lokalisation. Dtsch Med Wochenschr 97: 840–842
8. Barrett GM (1974) Hypotension after percutaneous liver biopsy. Lancet I: 624
9. Berg JW, Robbinson GF (1962) A late look at the safety of aspiration biopsy. Cancer 15: 826–827
10. Bergmann L (1954) Der Ultraschall. Hirzel, Stuttgart
11. Blady JV (1939) Aspiration biopsy of tumors in obscure or difficult locations under roentgenoscopic guidance. AJR 42: 515–524
12. Bönhof JA, Stapff M, Böhnhof B, Kremer H, Zöllner N, Lienhart P (1983) Das Bogenartefakt in der B-Bild-Sonographie. CT-Sonographie 3: 133–137
13. Bordas JM, Bru C, Bruguera M (1974) Hypotension and bradycardia after liver biopsy. Lancet I: 875
14. Born M, Wolf E (1970) Principles of optics. Pergamon, Oxford, p 452
15. Braun B, Dormeyer HH (1981) Ultrasonically guided fine needle aspiration biopsy of hepatic and pancreatic space-occupying lesions and percutaneous abscess drainage. Klin Wochenschr 59: 707–712
16. Buchborn R, Eigler J, Renner E (1970) Klinische Wertigkeit der Nierenbiopsie. Internist (Berlin) 11: 383–392
17. Büsing M (1984) Ergebnisse der ultraschallgeleiteten Feinnadelpunktion des Röntgendiagnostischen Zentralinstitutes des Universitätsspitals Zürich. Med Dissertation, Universität Zürich
18. Christoffersen P, Poll P (1970) Preoperative pancreas aspiration biopsy. Acta Pathol Microbiol Scand [suppl] 212: 28–32
19. Coley BL, Sharp GS, Ellis EB (1931) Diagnosis of bone tumors by aspiration. Am J Surg 13: 215–224
20. Coltori EA, Varela Diaz VM (1976) Survival of hydatid cysts after puncturing. Ann Parasitol Hum Comp 51: 647–652
21. Conn HO (1975) Liver biopsy in extrahepatic biliary obstruction and in other „contraindicated" disorders. Gastroenterology 68: 817–821
22. Conn HO (1974) Intrahepatic hematoma after liver biopsy. Gastroenterology 67: 375–381
23. Conrad MR, Sanders RC, Mascardo AD (1977) Perinephritic abscess aspiration using ultrasound guidance. AJR 128: 459–464
24. De Ford JW (1974) Acute transient hypotension following percutaneous liver biopsy. Lancet I: 741

25. Desai SG, Woodruff LM (1974) Carcinoma of prostate. Local extension following perineal needle biopsy. Urology 3: 87–88
26. Ditscherlein G (1969) Morphologische Folgen der Nierenpunktion. Tierexperimentelle und humanpathologische Befunde. Springer, Berlin Heidelberg New York (Experimentelle Medizin, Pathologie und Klinik, Bd 29)
27. Dittrich P von, zur Nedden D, Klima G (1982) Der Wert der Computertomographie bei der perkutanen Nierenbiopsie und Versuche zur Vermeidung der postpunktionellen Blutung. Z Urol Nephrol 75: 301–305
28. Dussik KT (1942) Über die Möglichkeit, hochfrequente mechanische Schwingungen als diagnostisches Hilfsmittel zu verwerten. Z Neurol Psychiatr 174: 153–168
29. Dussik KT, Dussik F, Wyt L (1947) Auf dem Wege zur Hyperphonographie des Gehirns. Wien Med Wochenschr 97: 425–429
30. Einighammer HJ, Hauke R (1982) Zum Problem der Erkennung von Punktionsnadeln im Ultraschallbild. Ultraschalldiagnostik '82, Bern. Thieme, Stuttgart New York, S. 88–90
31. Engelhart GJ, Blauenstein UW (1972) Ultraschalldiagnostik am Oberbauch. Schattauer, Stuttgart New York
32. Engzell U, Jakobsson PÅ, Sigurdson Å, Zajicek J (1971) Investigation on tumor spread in connection with aspiration biopsy. Acta Radiol [Diagn] (Stockh) 10: 385–398
33. Engzell U, Jakobsson PÅ, Sigurdson Å, Zajicek J (1971) Aspiration biopsy of metastatic carcinoma in lymph node of the neck. A review of 1101 consecutive cases. Acta Otolaryngol (Stockh) 72: 138
34. Esposti PL, Franzén J Zajicek J (1968) The aspiration biopsy smear. In: Koss LG (ed) Diagnostic cytology and its histopathologic bases, vol 2. Lippincott, Philadelphia, pp 565–596
35. Evans WK, Ho CS, McLoughlin MJ, Tao LC (1981) Fatal necrotizing pancreatitis following fine-needle aspiration biopsy of the pancreas. Radiology 141: 61–62
36. Falchuk KR (1974) Hypotension after percutaneous liver biopsy. Lancet I: 624
37. Feigenbaum H (1976) Echocardiography, 2nd edn. Lea & Febiger, Philadelphia
38. Ferguson RS (1930) Prostatic neoplasms. Their diagnosis by needle puncture and aspiration. Am J Surg 9: 507–511
39. Ferrucci JT, Wittenberg J, Margolies MN, Carey RW (1979) Malignant seeding of the tract after thin-needle aspiration biopsy. Radiology 130: 345–346
40. Ferrucci JT, Wittenberg J, Mueller PR, Simeone JF, Harbin WP, Kirkpatrick RH, Taft PD (1980) Diagnosis of abdominal malignancy by radiologic fine-needle aspiration biopsy. AJR 13: 323–330
41. Floyd KM (1974) Ethics of renal biopsy. Ann Intern Med 80: 117–118
42. Fornage BD, Touche DH, Deglaire M, Faroux M-JC, Simatos A (1983) Real-time ultrasound-guided prostatic biopsy using a new transrectal linear-array probe. Radiology 146: 547–548
43. Frable WJ (1976) Thin-needle aspiration biopsy. A personal experience with 469 cases. Am J Clin Pathol 65: 168–182
44. Frank H, Leodolter I (1966) Praktische Erfahrungen mit der ambulanten Leberbiopsie. Wien Klin Wochenschr 78: 756–758
45. Franzén S, Zajicek J (1968) Aspiration biopsy in diagnosis of palpable lesions of the breast. Acta Radiol 7: 241
46. Franzén S, Giertz G, Zajicek J (1960) Cytological diagnosis of prostatic tumours by transrectal aspiration biopsy. A preliminary report. Br J Urol 32: 193–196
47. Fraser RA, Leary FJ (1973) Ureterocutaneous fistula following percutaneous renal biopsy. J Urol 109: 931–933
48. Fritzsche P, Moorhead JD, Axford PD, Torrey RR (1981) Urologic application of angiographic guide wire and catheter techniques. J Urol 125: 774–780
49. Garret M, Herbsman H, Fierst S (1977) Cytologic diagnosis of echinococcosis. Acta Cytol (Baltimore) 21: 553–554
50. Gebel M (1982) Letaler Ausgang einer Leberpunktion bei Hämangiom (persönliche Mitteilung)
51. Gledhill EY, Spriggs JB, Binford CH (1949) Needle aspiration in diagnosis of lung carcinoma; report of experience with 75 aspirations. Am J Clin Pathol 19: 235–242
52. Goldberg BB, Pollack HH (1972) Ultrasonic aspiration transducer. Radiology 102: 187–189

53. Goldberg BB, Ziskin MC (1973) Echo patterns with an aspiration ultrasonic transducer. Invest Radiol 8: 78–83
54. Goldin AR (1977) Percutaneous ureteral splinting. Urology 10: 165–168
55. Goodwin WE, Casey WC, Woolf W (1955) Percutaneous trocar (needle) nephrostomy in hydronephrosis. JAMA 891–894
56. Göttinger H, Schilling A, Schüller J, Marx FJ (1980) Die perkutane Nierenfistelung – Indikation, Technik und Nachsorge. Med Welt 31: 1704–1708
57. Grabstald H, McPhee M (1973) Nephrostomy and the cancer patient. South Med J 66: 217–220
58. Grant AP, Robb JJ (1973) Liver biopsy in general medicine. Ten years experience. Ulster Med J 42: 179–183
59. Grundmann E (1979) Keine Metastasenförderung durch Biopsien. Dtsch Ärztebl 76: 699–702
60. Grundmann R, Eitenmüller J, Pichlmaier H (1981) Zur Indikation der verschiedenen Operationsverfahren bei Leberechinococcus. Chirurg 52: 332–337
61. Günther R, Alken P, Altwein JE (1978) Perkutane Nephropyelostomie-Anwendungsmöglichkeiten und Ergebnisse. ROEFO 128: 720–726
62. Günther R, Alken P, Altwein JE (1978) Ureterobstruktion: Perkutane transrenale Uretersplintung. Aktuel Urol 9: 195–199
63. Guthrie CG (1921) Gland puncture as a diagnostic measure. Bull Johns Hopkins Hosp 32: 266
64. Haaga JR, Alfidi RJ (1976) Precise biopsy localization by computed tomography. Radiology 118: 603–607
65. Harzmann R, Haacke C, Bichler KH (1981) Neuentwicklung eines Einmalsystems für die perkutane Nephrostomie. Urologe [Ausg A] 20: 63–67
66. Heckemann R, Heimann H, Meyer-Schwickerath M, Paar D, Eickenberg HU (1982) Ultraschallgeführte Nierenzysten-Punktion. ROEFO 137: 26–30
67. Heckemann R, Seidel KJ (1982) In-vitro und In-vivo-Darstellungen von Punktionsinstrumenten im sonographischen Echtzeitbild, 1: Punktionsnadeln. Ultraschall 3: 18–23
68. Hirschfeld H (1912) Über isolierte aleukämische Lymphadenose der Haut. Z Krebsforsch 11: 397–407
69. Hjelmroth HE (1980) Puncture needles and ultrasonic wave propagation in ultrasonically guided puncture technique. In: Holm HH, Kristensen JK (eds) Ultrasonically guided puncture technique. Munksgaard, Copenhagen, pp 25–28
70. Hodenak N, Lees WR, Pereira J, Beilby JOW, Cotton PB (1982) Ultrasound – guides percutaneous fine-needle aspiration cytology in pancreatic cancer. Br Med J 285: 1183–1184
71. Holm H, Gammelgaard J (1981) Ultrasonically guided precise needle placement in the prostate and the seminal vesicles. J Urol 125: 385–387
72. Holm HH, Hancke S, Gronwall S, Krag Jacobsen G (1982) Interventional Ultrasound. In: Lerski RA, Morley P (eds) Ultrasound 1982. Kongressband 3. WFUMB-Convention, Brighton. Pergamon, Oxford, pp 429–437
73. Holm HH, Kristensen JK, Rasmussen SN, Northeved A, Barlebo H (1972) Ultrasound as a guide in percutaneous puncture technique. Ultrasonics 10: 83–86
74. Hounsfield GN (1973) Computerized transverse axial scanning (tomography): Part 1. Description of system. Br J Radiol 46: 1016–1022
75. House AJS, Thomson KR (1977) Evaluation of a new transthoracic needle for biopsy of benign and malignant lung lesions. AJR 129: 215–220
76. Hricak H, Crůz C, Romanski R et al. (1982) Renal parenchymal disease: Sonographic-histologic correlation. Radiology 144: 141–147
77. Iversen R, Brun C (1951) Aspiration biopsy of kidney. Am J Med 11: 324–330
78. Iversen P, Roholm K (1939) On aspiration biopsy of the liver, with remarks on its diagnostic significance. Acta Med Scand 102: 1–16
79. Izumi S, Tamaki S, Natori H, Kira S (1982) Ultrasonically guided aspiration needle biopsy in disease of the chest. Am Rev Respir Dis 125: 460–464
80. Jacobson ES (1973) A case of secondary echinococcosis diagnosed by cytologic examination of pleural fluid and needle biopsy of the pleura. Acta Cytol (Baltimore) 17: 76–79
81. Jensen F (1980) Physical principles for ultrasonically guided puncture. In: Holm HH, Kristensen JK (eds) Ultrasonically guided puncture technique. Munksgaard, Copenhagen, pp 21–24

82. Jonatha W (1974) Amniozentese in der Frühschwangerschaft unter Sichtkontrolle mit Ultraschall. Elektromedica 3
83. Kark RM, Muehrcke RC (1954) Biopsy of kidney in prone position. Lancet I: 1047-1049
84. Kasai Y, Koshino I, Kawanishi N, Sakamoto H, Sasaki E, Kumagai M (1980) Alveolar echinococcosis of the liver. Studies on 60 operated cases. Ann Surg 191: 145-152
85. Klahn H, Waldthaler A, Voeth C, Ottenjann R (1983) Perkutane, ultraschallgezielte Feinnadelpunktionen (Leber, Pankreas und Darm) und ultraschallgezielte Pankreasgangpunktionen. Dtsch Med Wochenschr 108: 1503-1507
86. Kline TS, Neal HS (1973) Needle biopsy, a pilot study. JAMA 224: 1143-1146
87. Knoflach P, Judmaier G, Reiner A, Mikuz G (1983) Ultraschallgezielte Feinnadelpunktion. Wien Med Wochenschr 133: 514-519
88. Kollwitz AA (1961) Eine Übersicht über 5700 perkutane Nierenbiopsien. Med Klin 56: 726-731
89. Kratochwil A (1977) Ultraschalldiagnostik in der Inneren Medizin, Chirurgie und Urologie. Thieme, Stuttgart
90. Krautkrämer J, Krautkrämer H (1980) Werkstoffprüfung mit Ultraschall. Springer, Berlin Heidelberg New York
91. Kristensen JK, Holm HH, Rasmussen SN, Barbelo H (1972) Ultrasonically guided percutaneous puncture of renal masses. Scand J Urol Nephrol [Suppl] 15: 49
92. Labardini MM, Nesbit RM (1967) Perineal extension of adenocarcinoma of the prostata gland after punch biopsy. J Urol 97: 891-893
93. Lebert H (1851) Traité pratique des maladies cancéreuses et des affections curables confondues avec le cancer. Baillière, Paris
94. Lee Y-TN (1974) Maligmant melanoma: To biopsy or not to biopsy. CA 24: 104-105
95. Leiter E, Gribetz D, Cohen S (1972) Arterio-venous fistula after percutaneous needle biopsy-surgical repair with preservation of renal function. N Engl J Med 287: 971-972
96. Linder H (1971) Das Risiko der perkutanen Leberbiopsie. Med Klin 66: 926-929
97. Livraghi T, Damascelli B, Lombardi C, Spagnoli I (1983) Risk in fine-needle abdominal biopsy. J Clin Ultrasound 11: 77-81
98. Lopes Cardozo P (1979) Atlas of clinical cytology. S'Hertogenbosch: Targa. Lippincott, Philadelphia, Chemie-Verlag, Weinheim
99. Lüdin H (1955) Die Organpunktion in der klinischen Diagnostik. Gefahren der Leberpunktion. Karger, Basel New York, S 121-125
100. Ludwig GD, Struthers FW (1949) Consideration underlying the use of ultrasound to detect gallstones and foreign bodies in tissue. Proj. N.M. 004:001. US Naval Med Res Inst 4: 1-27
101. Lutz H, Weidenhiller S, Rettenmaier G (1973) Ultraschallgezielte Feinnadelbiopsie der Leber. Schweiz Med Wochenschr 103: 1030-1033
102. Manitz G (1974) Offene oder perkutane Nierenbiopsie aus der Sicht des Internisten. Urologe [Ausg A] 13: 124-126
103. Martin HE, Ellis EB (1930) Biopsy by needle puncture and aspiration. Ann Surg 92: 169-181
104. Martin HE, Stewart FW (1936) Advantages and limitations of aspiration biopsy. AJR 35: 245-247
105. Marx FJ (1981) Perkutane Nephrostomie: Ballonkatheter-System. Perkutane Eingriffe am oberen Harntrakt. Tübinger Symposium (7.11.1981)
106. Mazer MJ, Le Veen RF, Call JE, Wolg G, Baltaxe HA (1979) Permanent percutaneous antegrade ureteral stent placement without transurethral assistance. Urology 14: 413-419
107. McDicken WN (1976) Diagnostic ultrasonics: Principles and use of instruments. Clowes, London Beccles Colchester, p 256
108. McGill DB (1981) Predicting hemorrhage after liver biopsy. Editorial. Dig Dis Sci 26: 285-387
109. Menghini G (1970) Current concepts: One-second biopsy of the liver-problems of its clinical application. N Engl J Med 283: 582-585
110. Menghini G (1957) Un effettivo progresso nella tecnica della puntura-biopsia del fegato. 7: 756-773
111. Milner LB, Ryan K, Gullo J (1979) Fatal intrathoracic hemorrhage after percutaneous aspiration lung biopsy. AJR 132: 280-281
112. Mitty HA, Efremidis SC, Yeh HC (1981) Impact of fine-needle biopsy on management of patients with carcinoma of the pancreas. AJR 137: 1119-1121

154

113. Moeschlin S (1947) Die Milzpunktion. Schwabe, Basel
114. Montali G, Solbiati L, Croce F, Ierace I, Ravetto C (1982) Fine-needle aspiration biopsy of liver focal lesions ultrasonically guided with a real-time probe. Report on 126 cases. Br J Radiol 55: 717–723
115. Müller J (1838) Über den feineren Bau und die Formen der krankhaften Geschwülste. Reimer, Berlin
116. Muth RG (1965) The safety of percutaneous renal biopsy: An analysis of 500 consecutive cases. J Urol 94: 1–3
117. Nordenström B, Sinner WN (1978) Needle biopsies of pulmonary lesions. Precaution and management of complications. ROEFO 129: 414–418
118. O'Conor VJ, Bergan JR, Bergan JJ (1973) Surgical repair in a solitary kidney of a large intrarenal arteriovenous fistula resulting from needle biopsy. J Urol 109: 934–937
119. Oeser H (1974) Krebsbekämpfung: Hoffnung und Realität. Thieme, Stuttgart, S 32–33
120. Olbing H (1979) Nierenbiopsie bei Kindern. Springer, Berlin Heidelberg New York, S 1–2
121. Otho M (1983) (persönliche Mitteilung; Zürich)
122. Otto R (1980) Ultraschallgesteuerte Organpunktion unter direkter Sicht. Tumorbiopsie, Amniocentese, Kombination mit Röntgenuntersuchungen. Acta Medicotech 28: 227–229
123. Otto R (1982) Results of 1000 fine needle punctures guided unter real-time sonographic control. J Belge Radiol 65: 193–199
124. Otto RC (1983) Indikationen für ultraschallgeleitete Eingriffe unter permanenter Sicht. 2. Therapeutische Punktionen. Ultraschall 4: 77–80
125. Otto RC (1980) Aktuelle Röntgendiagnostik im Kampf gegen den Brustkrebs. Huber, Bern Stuttgart Wien, S 126–127
126. Otto R, Deyhle P (1979) Ultraschallgezielte Feinnadelpunktion unter permanenter Sichtkontrolle. Vorläufige Ergebnisse. Dtsch Med Wochenschr 104: 1667–1669
127. Otto R, Deyhle P (1980) Guided puncture under real-time sonographic control. Radiology 134: 784–785
128. Otto R, Hauri D, Meier J, Wellauer J (1982) Perkutane ultraschallgeleitete Nephrostomie unter permanenter Sicht. ROEFO 137: 665–668
129. Otto R, Meier J, Buchmann P (1982) Perkutane Cholezysto- und Cholangiographie. Dtsch Med Wochenschr 107: 15–20
130. Otto R, Weihe W, Burger HR (1984) Zur Beurteilung der ultraschallgezielten Feinnadelpunktion. Experimentelle Untersuchungen am Hund. Dtsch Tierärztl Wochenschr 91: 178–182
131. Otto R, Woodtli W, Ammann R (1982) Sonographie versus CT bei Lebermanifestationen der Echinokokkose. Dtsch Med Wochenschr 107: 1717–1721
132. Perloff LJ, Jenis EH, Goodloe S, Light JA, Spees EK (1973) Value of one-hour renal-allograft biopsy. Lancet II: 1294–1295
133. Permanetter W, Bassermann R, Denecke H (1981) Diagnose des Echinokokkus cysticus mit cytologischer Methode. Chirurg 52: 187–189
134. Perrault J, McGill DB, Ott BJ, Taylor WF (1978) Liver biopsy: Complications in 1000 inpatients and outpatients. Gastroenterology 74: 103–106
135. Pohlmann R (1939) Über die Absorption des Ultraschalls im menschlichen Gewebe und ihre Abhängigkeit von der Frequenz. Phys Z 40: 159–161
136. Portier A, Janssen B, Dreyfus G, Robineau M (1981) Rupture d'un kyste hydatique du foie sans effraction de la membrane proligère. Nouv Presse Med 10: 176
137. Rettenmaier G (1976) Sonographischer Oberbauchstatus. Aussagefähigkeit und Indikationen der Ultraschall-Schnittbilduntersuchung des Oberbauchs. Internist (Berlin) 17: 549–564
138. Robbins GF, Brothers JH, Eberhart WF, Quan S (1954) Is aspiration biopsy of breast cancer dangerous to the patient? Cancer 7: 774–778
139. Rogers CA, Sharp HC (1974) Complications of percutaneous liver biopsy. Lancet I: 931
140. Rosenblatt R, Kutcher R, Moussouris HF, Schrieber K, Koss LG (1982) Sonographically guided fine-needle aspiration of liver lesions. JAMA 248: 1639–1641
141. Rutner AB, Fucilla I (1979) Percutaneous pigtail nephrostomy. Presented at the American Urologic Association. Ind Tuscon, Arizona, pp 18–22
142. Sagar SJ, Kaye MB (1973) Systemic infection following needle biopsy of the kidney. J Urol 109: 930

143. Saitoh M, Watanabe H, Ohe H (1980) Ultrasonic real-time guidance for percutaneous puncture in urology. In: Holm HH, Kristensen JK (eds) Ultrasonically guided puncture technique. Munksgaard, Copenhagen, pp 55–60
144. Sandberg AA, Moore GE, Schubarg JR (1959) „Atypical" cells in the blood of cancer patients; differentiation from tumour cells. J Natl Cancer Inst 22: 555–565
145. Sargent N, Turner AF, Gordonson J, Schwinn CP, Pashky O (1974) Percutaneous pulmonary needle biopsy. Report of 350 patients. AJR 122: 758–768
146. Sbarounis CN, Toubouras M, Mikrou J, Kappas A, Lazarides DP (1981) Die operative Behandlung des Einbruchs des Echinokokkus cysticus der Leber in die Gallengänge. Chirurg 52: 445–449
147. Schläpfer E (1948) Über angebliche körperliche Unverletzlichkeit. Schweiz Med Wochenschr 78: 352–354
148. Schnyder PA, Candardjis G, Anderegg A (1981) Peritonitis after thin-needle aspiration biopsy of an abscess. AJR 137: 1271–1272
149. Schüller J, Walther V, Schmeller N, Chaussy C (im Druck) Neues perkutanes Nephrostomie-Set zur ultraschallgeführten Punktion. Aktuel Urol
150. Schütterle G, Fritsch H (1965) Tödliche Komplikationen nach Nierenblindpunktion. Med Klin 60: 184–189
151. Schwerk WB, Schmitz-Moormann P (1980) Sonographisch gezielte perkutane transperitoneale Aspirationsbiopsie raumfordernder Pankreasprozesse. Dtsch Med Wochenschr 105: 1019–1023
152. Schwerk WB, Schmitz-Moormann P (1981) Ultrasonically guided fine-needle biopsies in neoplastic liver disease: Cytohistologic diagnoses and echo pattern of lesions. Cancer 48: 1469–1477
153. Scotto J, Opolon P, Etévé J, Vergoz D, Thomas M, Caroli J (1973) Liver biopsy and prognosis in acute liver failure. Gut 14: 927–933
154. Servinc E, Özer H, Alp Niron E (1980) Hydatid cyst of liver: Ultrasonic classification and a new approach to the diagnosis. In: Conference on ultrasonically guided puncture, Herlev, Copenhagen 10.–12.9. 1980 (Abstracts 34)
155. Sherlock S (1962) Needle biopsy of the liver: A review. J Clin Pathol 15: 291–304
156. Sinner WN (ed) (1982) Needle biopsy and transbronchial biopsy. Thieme, Stuttgart New York, pp 50–53
157. Sinner WN (1980) Riskfactors in percutaneous transthoracic needle biopsy. ROEFO 132: 363–368
158. Sinner WN, Zajicek J (1976) Implantation metastasis after percutaneous transthoracic needle aspiration biopsy. Acta Radiol. [Diagn] (Stockh) 17: 473–480
159. Šlais J, Mádle A, Vanka K, Jelínek F, Černík V, Průchová M, Jindra J (1979) Alveolar hydatidosis (echinococcosis) diagnosed by liver puncture biopsy. Čas Lek Cesk 118: 472–475
160. Smith EH (im Druck) The hazards of fine-needle aspiration biopsy. Ultrasound Med Biol
161. Spitzer A (1979) Indikationen für die Nierenbiopsie bei Kindern mit nephrotischen Syndromen, Glomerulonephritis und Proteinurie/Hämaturie. In: Olbing H (Hrsg) Nierenbiopsie bei Kindern. Springer, Berlin Heidelberg New York, S 33–53
162. Spratt JS, Donegan WL (1967) Cancer of the breast. Saunders, Philadelphia London
163. Stahel R (1939) Diagnostische Drüsenpunktion. Thieme, Leipzig
164. Sullivan S, Watson WC (1974) Acute transient hypotension as complication of percutaneous liver biopsy. Lancet I: 389–390
165. Takada E, Morikubo H, Tsuchidate M, Shida S, Tanaka M (1980) Artefacts of electric linear scanner. ISUM Proc 55: 101
166. Tsuchiya Y (1969) A new and safer method of percutaneous transhepatic cholangiography (in Japanisch). Jpn J Gastroenterol 66: 438–455
167. Von Schreeb T, Arner O, Skovsted G, Wikstad N (1967) Renal adenocarcinoma. Is there a risk of spreading tumour cells in diagnostic puncture? Scand J Urol Nephrol 1: 270–276
168. Ward GR (1913) The blood in cancer with bone metastases. Lancet I: 676
169. Weens HS, Florence TJ (1954) The diagnosis of hydronephrosis by percutaneous renal puncture. J Urol 72: 589–595
170. Wells PNT (1977) Biomedical ultrasonics. Academic Press, London

171. Westcott JL (1980) Direct percutaneous needle aspiration of localized pulmonary lesions: Results in 422 patients. Radiology 137: 31–35
172. White RHR, Jivani SKM (1974) Evaluation of a disposible needle for renal biopsy in children. Clin Nephrol 2: 120–122
173. Wickboom I (1954) Pyelography after direct puncture of the renal pelvis. Acta Radiol [Diagn] (Stockh) 41: 505–512
174. Wilbur RD, Foulk WT (1967) Percutaneous liver biopsy. JAMA 202: 147–149
175. Wild JJ, Neal D (1951) Use of high frequency ultrasonic waves for detecting changes of texture in living tissues. Lancet I: 655–657
176. Wildhirt E, Möller E (1981) Erfahrungen bei nahezu 20000 Leberblindpunktionen. Med Klin 76: 254–256
177. Wimmer B, Kauffmann G, Sinagowitz E (1980) Perkutane Nephropyelostomie: Kombination sonographischer und röntgenologischer Technik. Röntgenblätter 33: 147–155
178. Wolinsky H, Lischner MW (1969) Needle tract implantation of tumor after percutaneous lung biopsy. Ann Intern Med 71: 359–362
179. Yamauchi H, Hopper J, McCormack K, Lambert K (1960) Hypovolemia in the nephrotic syndrome – a contraindication to renal biopsy. N Engl J Med 263: 1012–1014
180. Zajicek J (1974) Aspiration biopsy cytology, vol 4, part 1: Cytology of supradiaphragmatic organs. Karger, Basel München Paris London New York Sydney
181. Zajicek J (1979) Aspiration biopsy cytology, part 2: Cytology of infradiaphragmatic organs. Karger, Basel München Paris London New York Sydney (Monographs in clinical cytology, vol 7)
182. Zamcheck N, Klausenstock O (1953) Needle biopsy of the liver. II. The risk of needle biopsy. N Engl J Med 249: 1062–1069
183. Zelman S (1954) Fatal hemorrhage following needle biopsy in uremia. JAMA 154: 997–1000

Subject Index